Clinical Pocket Manual™

Signs and Symptoms

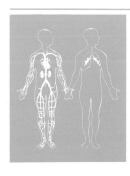

NURSING85 BOOKS™
SPRINGHOUSE CORPORATION
SPRINGHOUSE, PENNSYLVANIA

D1611681

Clinical Pocket Manual™ Series

PROGRAM DIRECTOR
Jean Robinson

CLINICAL DIRECTOR
Barbara McVan, RN

ART DIRECTOR
John Hubbard

EDITORIAL MANAGER
Susan R. Williams

EDITORS
Lisa Z. Cohen
Kathy E. Goldberg
Virginia P. Peck

CLINICAL EDITORS
Joan E. Mason, RN, EdM
Diane Schweisguth, RN, BSN

COPY SUPERVISOR
David R. Moreau

DESIGNER
Maria Errico

PRODUCTION COORDINATOR
Susan Powell-Mishler

Material in this book was adapted from the following series: Nurse's Reference Library, Nursing Photobook, New Nursing Skillbook, Nursing Now, and Nurse's Clinical Library.

CPM4-011085

Library of Congress Cataloging-in-Publication Data

Main entry under title:

Signs and symptoms.

  (Clinical pocket manual)
  "Nursing85 books."
  Includes index.
  1. Diagnosis—Handbooks, manuals, etc.
  2. Nursing—Handbooks, manuals, etc.
  3. Symptomatology—Handbooks, manuals, etc.
  I. Series. [DNLM: 1. Diagnosis—handbooks.
2. Nursing Process—methods—handbooks.
WB 39 S578]
RT48.S55 1985   616.07′5   85-17295
ISBN 0-87434-005-5

CONTENTS

Nursing85 Books™

CLINICAL POCKET MANUAL™ SERIES
Diagnostic Tests
Emergency Care
Fluids and Electrolytes
Signs and Symptoms
Cardiovascular Care
Respiratory Care
Critical Care
Neurologic Care

NURSING NOW™ SERIES
Shock
Hypertension
Drug Interactions
Cardiac Crises
Respiratory Emergencies
Pain

NURSE'S CLINICAL LIBRARY™
Cardiovascular Disorders
Respiratory Disorders
Endocrine Disorders
Neurologic Disorders
Renal and Urologic Disorders
Gastrointestinal Disorders
Neoplastic Disorders
Immune Disorders

NURSING PHOTOBOOK™ SERIES
Providing Respiratory Care
Managing I.V. Therapy
Dealing with Emergencies
Giving Medications
Assessing Your Patients
Using Monitors
Providing Early Mobility
Giving Cardiac Care
Performing GI Procedures
Implementing Urologic Procedures
Controlling Infection
Ensuring Intensive Care
Coping with Neurologic Disorders
Caring for Surgical Patients
Working with Orthopedic Patients
Nursing Pediatric Patients
Helping Geriatric Patients
Attending Ob/Gyn Patients
Aiding Ambulatory Patients
Carrying Out Special Procedures

NURSE'S REFERENCE LIBRARY®
Diseases
Diagnostics
Drugs
Assessment
Procedures
Definitions
Practices
Emergencies
Signs and Symptoms

NURSE REVIEW™ SERIES
Cardiac Problems
Respiratory Problems

Nursing85 DRUG HANDBOOK™

Heart Failure: Signs and Symptoms

As a rule, signs and symptoms of left heart failure are pulmonary; those of right heart failure are systemic. Read the following for details on how signs and symptoms differ.

LEFT HEART FAILURE

- Elevated blood pressure
- Paroxysmal nocturnal dyspnea
- Dyspnea on exertion
- Orthopnea
- Bronchial wheezing
- Hypoxia
- Respiratory acidosis
- Crackles
- Cough with frothy pink sputum
- Cyanosis or pallor
- Third or fourth heart sounds
- Palpitations, dysrhythmias, tachycardia
- Elevated pulmonary artery and pulmonary capillary wedge pressures
- Pulsus alternans
- Oliguria

RIGHT HEART FAILURE

- Weakness, fatigue, dizziness, syncope
- Hepatomegaly, with or without pain
- Ascites
- Dependent pitting peripheral edema
- Jugular vein distention
- Hepatojugular reflux
- Oliguria
- Dysrhythmias, tachycardia
- Elevated central venous/right atrial pressure
- Nausea, vomiting, anorexia, abdominal distention
- Weight gain
- Splenomegaly (uncommon)

How to Intervene

If your patient's congestive heart failure becomes an emergency, intervene quickly and purposefully, using the priorities outlined below.
- Assess airway patency, and provide respiratory support, possibly mechanical ventilation, as necessary and ordered.
- Alert the doctor and other unit nurses.

- Administer oxygen.
- Position your patient to decrease venous return and relieve dyspnea.
- Start an I.V. for drug therapy.
- Run a 12-lead EKG.
- Obtain blood specimens for diagnostic tests.
- Monitor vital signs regularly.

Conditions of Reduced Myocardial Perfusion

ANGINA PECTORIS

Chief complaints
• *Chest pain:* may be dull or burning, or described as pressure, tightness, heaviness; builds and fades gradually; may be in abdomen; may radiate to jaw, teeth, face, left arm, neck, shoulders, upper abdomen, or back
• *Dyspnea:* possible, with sense of constriction around larynx or upper trachea
• *Fatigue:* absent
• *Irregular heartbeat:* may be present; patient complains of palpitations or skipped beats
• *Peripheral changes:* none

History
• Risk factors include family history of coronary artery disease, arteriosclerotic heart disease, cerebrovascular accident, diabetes, gout, hypertension, renal disease, obesity caused by excessive carbohydrate and saturated fat intake, smoking, lack of exercise, stress (Type A personality).
• Higher incidence in men over age 40; lower incidence in women prior to menopause.
• Precipitating factors include exertion, stress, cold or hot weather, and emotional excitement.

Physical examination
• Inspection reveals patient anxiety and diaphoresis.
• Palpation reveals tachycardia.
• Auscultation reveals change in blood pressure, possibly hypertension, especially during anginal attack; transient crackles associated with congestive heart failure; paradoxical splitting of S_2 possible.

Diagnostic studies
• EKG may be within normal limits, show depressed ST segments during ischemic attack, or show an atrioventricular conduction defect.
• Thallium stress imaging or stress EKG may show ischemic areas.
• Arteriogram reveals narrowing of coronary blood vessels.

Angina types
In general, angina is either stable or unstable. In stable angina, the frequency, duration, time of onset, and precipitating factors are predictable. Discomfort from stable angina is mild and infrequent. Stable angina can become unstable.

In unstable angina, frequency, duration, time of onset, and precipitating factors are unpredictable. Consequently, it's more serious than stable angina.

Continued

Conditions of Reduced Myocardial Perfusion
Continued

ACUTE MYOCARDIAL
INFARCTION

Chief complaints
• *Chest pain:* sudden but not instantaneous onset of constricting, crushing, heavy weightlike chest pain occuring at any time—not relieved by nitroglycerin; located centrally and substernally, although not usually in left chest; may build rapidly or in waves to maximum intensity in a few minutes; may be accompanied by nausea and vomiting (may radiate to jaw, teeth, face, left arm, neck, shoulders, upper abdomen, or back
• *Dyspnea:* present; may be accompanied by orthopnea, cough, and wheezing
• *Fatigue:* present; indicated by weakness and apprehension
• *Irregular heartbeat:* may be present; patient complains of palpitations or skipped beats
• *Peripheral changes:* peripheral cyanosis, with decreased perfusion
History
• Risk factors same as in angina pectoris.
• Past medical history may include episodes of angina pectoris.
Physical examination
• Patient will have a fever after 24 hours.

• Inspection reveals anxiety, tenseness, sense of impending doom, nausea, vomiting, and possibly distended neck veins, sweating, pallor, cyanosis, and shock.
• Palpation reveals tachycardia or bradycardia and possibly a weak or irregular pulse.
• Auscultation reveals normal or decreased blood pressure, significant murmurs that may preexist or occur with ruptured septum or ruptured papillary muscle, diminished gallop rhythm, pericardial friction rub, and crackles.
• In severe attack, shock, decreased urinary output, pulmonary edema.
Diagnostic studies
• EKG at onset shows elevated ST segment, which then returns to baseline; T waves become symmetrically inverted; abnormal Q waves present; may also show dysrhythmias.
• WBC count shows leukocytosis on second day (lasts 1 week); erythrocyte sedimentation rate normal at first, rises on second or third day.
• Enzyme testing shows elevated creatine phosphokinase (CPK) and CPK-MB initially; then increased SGOT and LDH.

Conditions Affecting Pump Action

LEFT VENTRICULAR FAILURE

Chief complaints
- *Chest pain:* usually absent
- *Dyspnea:* present on exertion, accompanied by cough, orthopnea, paroxysmal nocturnal dyspnea; in advanced disease, present at rest
- *Fatigue:* present on exertion, accompanied by weakness
- *Irregular heartbeat:* may be present; patient may complain of rapid heart rate and skipped beats

History
- Patient uses pillow to prop self up for sleep; wakes up gasping for breath; must sit or stand for relief.
- History of present illness includes wheezing on inspiration and expiration (cardiac asthma), right upper abdominal pain or discomfort on exertion, daytime oliguria, nighttime polyuria, constipation (uncommon), anorexia, progressive weight gain, generalized edema, progressive weakness, fatigue, decreased mentation.
- Past medical history includes severe chronic congestive heart failure.

Physical examination
- Inspection reveals profuse sweating, pallor or cyanosis, frothy white or pink sputum, heaving apical impulse, hand veins that remain distended when patient puts hands above level of right atrium.
- Palpation reveals enlarged, diffuse, and sustained left ventricular impulse at precordium, displaced to left; pulsus alternans at peripheral pulses.
- Percussion reveals pleural fluid (indicated by dullness at lung bases) and decreased tactile fremitus.
- Auscultation reveals S_3 and S_4 sounds, possibly mitral and tricuspid regurgitation murmurs, accentuated pulmonary component of second sound, decreased or absent breath sounds, crackles (basilar rales) that don't clear with coughing.

Diagnostic studies
- Pulmonary artery and pulmonary capillary wedge pressures elevated.
- Central venous pressure elevated if condition has advanced to right ventricular failure or hypervolemia.
- EKG reflects heart strain or left ventricular enlargement, ischemia, and dysrhythmias.
- Chest X-ray reveals left ventricular enlargement and pulmonary venous congestion with alveolar and interstitial edema.
- Urinalysis shows proteinuria and casts.

Continued

Conditions Affecting Pump Action
Continued

RIGHT VENTRICULAR FAILURE

Chief complaints
- *Chest pain:* usually absent
- *Dyspnea:* respiratory distress secondary to pulmonary disease or advanced left ventricular failure
- *Fatigue:* in severe cases, weakness and mental aberration
- *Irregular heartbeat:* atrial dysrhythmias common
- *Peripheral changes:* dependent edema; begins in ankles but progresses to legs and genitalia; initially subsides at night, later does not; ascites; weight gain

History
- History of present illness includes anorexia; right upper abdominal pain or discomfort during exertion; nausea; and vomiting.
- Past medical history includes left ventricular failure, mitral stenosis, pulmonic valve stenosis, tricuspid regurgitation, pulmonary hypertension, chronic obstructive pulmonary disease.

Physical examination
- Inspection reveals lower sternal or left parasternal heave independent of apical impulse.
- Palpation and percussion reveal enlarged, tender, pulsating liver, with tricuspid regurgitation; abdomen fluid wave and shifting dullness; hepatojugular reflux, indicating jugular vein distention; tachycardia.
- Auscultation reveals right ventricular S$_3$ sound; murmur of tricuspid regurgitation.

Diagnostic studies
- Central venous pressure readings are elevated.

CONGESTIVE CARDIOMYOPATHIES

Chief complaints
- *Dyspnea:* paroxysmal nocturnal, accompanied by orthopnea
- *Fatigue:* present
- *Irregular heartbeat:* palpitations: Stokes-Adams attacks with conduction defects
- *Peripheral changes:* dry skin, extremity pain, edema, and ascites with right-sided failure

History
- Viral illness, alcoholism, chronic debilitating illnesses.

Physical examination
- Fever
- Signs of heart failure
- Palpation reveals displaced cardiac impulse to left; tachycardia.
- Auscultation reveals systolic murmur, S$_3$ sound, and postural hypotension.

Diagnostic studies
- EKG reveals nonspecific ST-T changes, decreased height of R wave; may show dysrhythmias and conduction defects.

Continued

Conditions Affecting Pump Action
Continued

CONGESTIVE
CARDIOMYOPATHIES
Continued

• Echocardiography and chest X-ray may help determine heart size.

HYPERTROPHIC
CARDIOMYOPATHIES

Chief complaints
• *Chest pain:* present; similar to angina pectoris; but unrelieved by nitroglycerin
• *Dyspnea:* present on exertion
• *Fatigue:* present; accompanied by dizziness and syncope
• *Irregular heartbeat:* may be present; patient may complain of palpitations or skipped beats
• *Peripheral changes:* peripheral edema (uncommon)
History
• Symptoms may be induced by high temperatures, pregnancy, exercise, standing suddenly, Valsalva's maneuver.
Physical examination
• Palpation reveals peripheral pulse with characteristic double impulse.
• Auscultation reveals systolic ejection murmur.
• Signs of mitral insufficiency, congestive heart failure; sudden death possible.

Diagnostic studies
• EKG reveals left ventricular hypertrophy, ST segment, and T wave abnormalities.
• Echocardiography shows increased thickness of the interventricular system and abnormal motion of the mitral valve.

PERICARDITIS

Chief complaints
• *Chest pain:* sudden onset; precordial or substernal; pleuritic; radiating to left neck, shoulder, back, or epigastrium; worsened by lying down or swallowing
• *Dyspnea:* usually absent; breathing may cause pain
• *Fatigue:* usually absent
• *Irregular heartbeat:* absent
• *Peripheral changes:* none
History
• Past medical history includes viral respiratory infection, recent pericardiotomy or myocardial infarction, disseminated lupus erythematosus, serum sickness, acute rheumatic fever, trauma, uremia, lymphoma, dissecting aorta.
• Most common in men between ages 20 and 50
Physical examination
• Fever: 100° to 103° F. (37.8° to 39.4° C.)
• Palpation reveals tachycardia.

Continued

Conditions Affecting Pump Action
Continued

PERICARDITIS
Continued

• Auscultation reveals pericardial friction rub.
Diagnostic studies
• EKG shows ST-T segment elevation in all leads; returns to baseline in a few days, with T wave inversion.
• Possibly atrial fibrillation

PERICARDITIS WITH EFFUSION

Chief complaints
• *Chest pain:* may be present as dull, diffuse, oppressive precordial or substernal distress; dysphagia
• *Dyspnea:* present; associated with cough that causes patient to lean forward for relief
• *Fatigue:* usually absent
• *Irregular heartbeat:* absent
• *Peripheral changes:* none
History
• Past medical history includes uremia, malignancy, connective tissue disorder, viral pericarditis.
Physical examination
• Inspection reveals distended neck veins.
• Palpation and percussion reveal tachycardia, enlarged area of cardiac dullness, apical beat that's within dullness border or not palpable.
• Auscultation reveals abnormal blood pressure and possibly peri-

cardial friction rub, and acute cardiac tamponade (inspiratory distention of neck veins, narrow pulse pressure, paradoxical pulse); may progress to shock.
Diagnostic studies
• EKG shows T waves flat, low diphasic or inverted leads, QRS voltage uniformly low.

SUBACUTE AND ACUTE BACTERIAL ENDOCARDITIS

Chief complaints
• *Chest pain:* pain also present in abdomen and, uncommonly, in flanks
• *Dyspnea:* present in approximately 50% of cases; depends on severity of disease or valve involved
• *Fatigue:* present, usually as malaise
• *Irregular heartbeat:* absent
• *Peripheral changes:* weight loss, heart failure symptoms
History
• Present or recent history includes acute infection, surgery or instrumentation, dental work, drug abuse, abortion, transurethral prostatectomy.
• Past medical history includes rheumatic, congenital, or atherosclerotic heart disease.
Physical examination
• Daily fever
• Inspection may reveal petechiae
Continued

Conditions Affecting Pump Action
Continued

BACTERIAL ENDOCARDITIS
Continued

on conjunctivae and palate buccal mucosa; with long-standing endocarditis, clubbed fingers and toes; splinter hemorrhages beneath nails; tender red nodules on finger and toe pads (Osler's nodes); pallor or yellow-brown tint to skin; oval, pale, retinal lesion around optic disk (seen with ophthalmoscope).
• Auscultation reveals sudden change in present heart murmur or development of new murmur and possibly signs of early heart failure or emboli.

Diagnostic studies
• Blood cultures determine causative organism.
• Echocardiography—particularly the two-dimensional (2-D) method—looks for vegetation on valves.

Treatment
The goal of treatment is to eradicate the infecting organism. Therapy should start promptly and continue over several weeks. Antibiotic selection is based on sensitivity studies of the infecting organism—or the probable organism, if blood cultures are negative. I.V. antibiotic therapy usually lasts about 4 weeks.

Supportive treatment includes bed rest, aspirin for fever and aches, and sufficient fluid intake. Severe valvular damage, especially aortic regurgitation or infection of cardiac prosthesis, may require corrective surgery if refractory heart failure develops.

RHEUMATIC FEVER (ACUTE)

Chief complaints
• *Chest pain:* absent
• *Dyspnea:* may be present
• *Fatigue:* malaise
• *Irregular heartbeat:* absent
• *Gastrointestinal:* weight loss
• *Other:* sore throat, pallor

History
• Recent history includes streptococcal infection of upper respiratory tract (in previous 4 weeks), anorexia.
• Past medical history includes migratory, gradual arthritis; recurrent epistaxis; "growing pains" in joints (arthralgia).
• Increased clumsiness

Physical examination
• Usually low-grade fever, with sinus tachycardia disproportional to fever level
• Inspection reveals erythema marginatum (ring- or crescent-shaped macular rash), subcutaneous nodules (uncommon except in children), swollen joints (arthritis), Sydenham's chorea.
• Palpation reveals enlarged heart, abdominal tenderness or pain.

Continued

Conditions Affecting Pump Action
Continued

RHEUMATIC FEVER (ACUTE)
Continued

• Auscultation reveals mitral or aortic diastolic murmurs, varying heart sound quality, and possibly gallop rhythm, dysrhythmias, and ectopic beats.

Diagnostic studies
• Erythrocyte sedimentation rate (ESR) and WBC count elevated.
• C-reactive protein elevated.
• Throat cultures positive for beta-hemolytic streptococci.
• Antistreptolysin titer elevated.
• Chest X-ray may show cardiac enlargement.
• Electrocardiogram shows PR greater than 0.2 seconds; may further define dysrhythmias.

Treatment
Effective management eradicates the streptococcal infection, relieves symptoms, and prevents recurrence, reducing the chance of permanent cardiac damage. During the acute phase, treatment includes penicillin or (for patients with penicillin hypersensitivity) erythromycin. Salicylates, such as aspirin, relieve fever and minimize joint swelling and pain; if carditis is present or salicylates fail to relieve pain and inflammation, corticosteroids may be used. Supportive treatment requires strict bed rest for about 5 weeks during the acute phase with active carditis, followed by a progressive increase in physical activity, depending on clinical and laboratory findings and the response to treatment.

To decrease joint pain, use lightweight clothing and a bed cradle. Do not perform massage or apply hot or cold packs.

After the acute phase subsides, a monthly I.M. injection of penicillin G benzathine or daily doses of oral sulfadiazine or penicillin G may be used to prevent recurrence.

Such preventive treatment usually continues for at least 5 years or until age 25. Congestive heart failure necessitates continued bed rest and diuretics. Severe mitral or aortic valvular dysfunction causing persistent congestive heart failure requires corrective valvular surgery, including commissurotomy (separation of the adherent, thickened leaflets of the mitral valve), valvuloplasty (repair of valve), or valve replacement (with prosthetic valve). Corrective valvular surgery is rarely necessary before late adolescence or early adulthood.

Conditions of Incompetent Peripheral Circulation

VARICOSE VEINS

Chief complaint
• *Peripheral changes:* aching discomfort or pain in legs; pigmentation and ulceration of distal leg; possibly edema

History
• History of present illness includes leg cramps at night that may be relieved by leg elevation, itching in vein regions, leg fatigue caused by periods of standing.
• Past medical history includes thrombophlebitis and family history of varicosities.

Physical examination
• Inspection reveals dilated, tortuous vessels in legs, visible when patient stands; brown pigmentation and thinning of skin above ankles; ulceration of distal leg; positive Trendelenburg's test.

Diagnostic studies
• None usually performed.

THROMBOPHLEBITIS

Chief complaints
• *Chest pain:* present with pulmonary embolism
• *Peripheral changes:* pain and swelling of affected extremity; if leg veins affected, pain may increase with walking

History
• Possible childbirth 4 to 14 days before onset
• History of present illness includes fracture, trauma, deep-vein surgery, cardiac disease, cerebrovascular accident, prolonged bed rest.
• Past medical history includes malignancy, shock, dehydration, anemia, obesity, chronic infection, use of oral contraceptives.
• In superficial vein thrombophlebitis, recent history includes superficial vein I.V. therapy with irritating solutions.

Physical examination
• Increased temperature and pulse
• In deep-vein involvement, inspection reveals cyanotic skin in affected area (with severe venous obstruction); pale and cool skin (with reflex arterial spasm).
• Palpation reveals warm affected leg, spasm and pain in calf muscles with dorsiflexion of foot (positive Homans' sign); veins are hard, thready, and sensitive to pressure.
• In superficial-vein involvement, inspection reveals induration, redness, tenderness along course of vein; possibly no clinical manifestations.

Diagnostic studies
• Ultrasound blood flow detector, thermography, and phlebography used to confirm diagnosis.

Continued

Conditions of Incompetent Peripheral Circulation
Continued

DISSECTING THORACIC AORTIC ANEURYSM

Chief complaints
- *Chest pain:* present; sudden and severe, radiating to back, abdomen, and hips
- *Dyspnea:* present
- *Peripheral changes:* absent

History
- Recent history may include seizures.
- Past medical history includes hypertension, arteriosclerosis, congenital heart disease, Marfan's syndrome, pregnancy, trauma

Physical examination
- Fever
- Dilated superficial veins on neck, arms, and chest.
- Palpation reveals unequal or diminished peripheral pulses, abdominal bruit.
- Auscultation reveals aortic diastolic murmur and murmurs over arteries.

Diagnostic studies
- Aortography shows size and extent of aneurysm.

ABDOMINAL AORTIC ANEURYSM

Chief complaint
- *Pain:* intermittent or persistent abdominal or low back pain radiating to flank and groin.

History
- Most common in men over age 50

Physical examination
- Inspection reveals subcutaneous ecchymosis in flank or groin.
- Palpation reveals pulsating midabdominal and upper abdominal mass.
- *Signs of shock (following rupture):* tachycardia, hypotension, weakness.

Diagnostic studies
- Aortography shows size of aneurysm.
- EKG, urinalysis, BUN evaluate renal and cardiac function.

RAYNAUD'S DISEASE AND RAYNAUD'S PHENOMENON

Chief complaints
- *Pain:* hands
- *Peripheral changes:* with Raynaud's disease: attacks of cyanosis, followed by pallor in fingers (rarely in thumbs or toes); coldness in hands without changes in pulses (radial or ulnar); redness, swelling, throbbing, and paresthesia during recovery, occurring when areas are warmed; numbness, stiffness, diminished sensation; with Raynaud's phenomenon: usually unilateral cyanosis, which may involve only one or two fingers

Continued

Conditions of Incompetent Peripheral Circulation
Continued

RAYNAUD'S DISEASE AND
RAYNAUD'S PHENOMENON
Continued

History
• Most common in females between puberty and age 40
• Precipitating factors include **emotional upsets** or cold
• Past history includes immunologic abnormalities.
• Family history of vasospastic diseases

• Raynaud's phenomenon may accompany cervical rib or carpal tunnel syndrome, scleroderma, systemic lupus erythematosus, frostbite, ergot poisoning.
Physical examination
• Inspection reveals dryness and atrophy of terminal fat pads of fingers, atrophy of fingernails, gangrene of fingertips.
Diagnostic studies
• None usually performed.

Treatment for Raynaud's Disease

Initially, treatment consists of avoidance of cold, mechanical, or chemical injury; cessation of smoking; and reassurance that symptoms are benign.

Encourage warm drinks and baths. Keep room temperature at or above 70° F. (21° C.). Carefully trim fingernails and apply lotions, emollients, and lubricants to the arms.

Since drug side effects, es-pecially from vasodilators, may be more bothersome than the disease itself, drug therapy is reserved for unusually severe symptoms. As ordered, administer drugs such as phenoxybenzamine or reserpine. Sympathectomy may be helpful when conservative modalities fail to prevent ischemic ulcers and thus may become necessary in less than 25% of these patients.

Conditions Affecting Valvular Function

TRICUSPID STENOSIS

Chief complaints
- *Chest pain:* usually absent
- *Dyspnea:* present in varying degrees
- *Fatigue:* present; often severe
- *Irregular heartbeat:* usually absent
- *Peripheral changes:* dependent peripheral edema

History
- More common in women than in men
- Past medical history includes mitral valve disease.

Physical examination
- Inspection may reveal olive skin.
- Palpation may reveal presystolic liver pulsation if in sinus rhythm; middiastolic thrill between lower left sternal border and apical impulse.
- Auscultation reveals diastolic rumbling murmur heard along lower left sternal border; normal blood pressure.

Diagnostic studies
- EKG shows wide, tall, peaked P waves; normal axis.
- Echocardiography may permit stenosis recognition.
- X-ray shows enlarged right atrium.
- Cardiac catheterization shows elevated central venous pressure and a pressure gradient across the tricuspid valve.

TRICUSPID REGURGITATION (INCOMPETENCE)

Chief complaints
- *Chest pain:* absent
- *Dyspnea:* present
- *Fatigue:* present; patient tires easily
- *Irregular heartbeat:* atrial fibrillation; usually not noticed by patient
- *Peripheral changes:* none

History
- Past medical history includes right ventricular failure, rheumatic fever, trauma, endocarditis, pulmonary hypertension.

Physical examination
- Palpation reveals right ventricular pulsation, systolic liver pulsation, and possibly systolic thrill at lower left sternal edge.
- Auscultation reveals blowing, coarse, or harsh systolic murmur heard along lower left sternal border; murmur sound increases on inspiration.

Diagnostic studies
- EKG usually shows atrial fibrillation.
- Cardiac catheterization dye flows backward from the right ventricle to the right atrium.

Continued

Conditions Affecting Valvular Function
Continued

AORTIC STENOSIS

Chief complaints
• *Chest pain:* present in severe stenosis
• *Dyspnea:* present, with coughing, on exertion; paroxysmal nocturnal; orthopnea
• *Fatigue:* usually present; syncope on exertion or change in position
• *Irregular heartbeat:* present, as palpitations occasionally

History
• More common in men than in women.
• Usually asymptomatic unless severe

Physical examination
• Inspection reveals apical impulse, localized and heaving, usually not laterally displaced.
• Palpation reveals sustained, localized, forceful apical impulse; systolic thrill over aortic area and neck vessels; small, slowly rising plateau pulse, best appreciated in carotid pulse.
• Late symptoms include weakness, debility, edema, ascites, and enlarged liver.
• Auscultation reveals harsh, rough, systolic ejection murmur in aortic area, radiating to the neck and apex; possibly systolic ejection click at aortic area just before murmur; paradoxical splitting of second sound with significant stenosis; normal or high diastolic blood pressure.

Diagnostic studies
• Electrocardiogram shows criteria for left ventricular hypertrophy; possibly complete heart block.
• X-ray examination and fluoroscopy may show calcified aortic valve, poststenotic dilation of ascending aorta (hyperactivity evident with fluoroscopy), left ventricular hypertrophy.
• Echocardiography may identify level of obstruction and a bicuspid aortic valve.
• Cardiac catheterization indicates the severity and location of the obstruction as well as left ventricular function.
• Angiocardiogram reveals degree of aortic stenosis and reduction of left ventricular capacity.

Continued

Conditions Affecting Valvular Function
Continued

AORTIC REGURGITATION (INCOMPETENCE)

Chief complaints

- *Chest pain:* angina pectoris
- *Dyspnea:* on exertion early in disease and at rest later in disease; paroxysmal nocturnal dyspnea; orthopnea and cough signal beginning of decompensation
- *Fatigue:* present; weakness if left ventricular failure present
- *Irregular heartbeat:* palpitations (signal beginning of decompensation); bounding pulse
- *Peripheral changes:* none

History

- Past medical history includes Reiter's syndrome, rheumatoid arthritis, psoriasis, rheumatic fever, syphilis, subacute bacterial endocarditis.

Physical examination

- Inspection reveals generalized skin pallor; strong, abrupt carotid pulsations; forceful apical impulse to left of left midclavicular line and downward; capillary pulsations.
- Palpation reveals sustained and forceful apical impulse, displaced to left and downward; rapidly rising and collapsing pulses.
- Auscultation reveals Austin Flint murmur that may be heard at apex; with diastolic pressure less than 60 mm Hg, possibly wide pulse pressure; systolic pressure may be normal or slightly elevated.
- In aortic insufficiency, auscultation reveals normal heart sounds; soft, blowing, diastolic murmur (heard over aortic area and apex; usually loudest along left sternal border).

Diagnostic studies

- Electrocardiogram shows evidence of left ventricular hypertrophy.
- X-ray examination shows enlarged left ventricle.
- Echocardiography demonstrates a flutter of the mitral valve during diastole and helps establish aortic valve incompetence.
- Cardiac catheterization and angiocardiography performed to exclude complicating lesions and to assess left ventricular function and magnitude of regurgitation.

Continued

Conditions Affecting Valvular Function
Continued

MITRAL STENOSIS

Chief complaints
- *Chest pain:* usually absent
- *Dyspnea:* present; shortness of breath; induced by exertion; may also occur during rest; orthopnea; paroxysmal nocturnal dyspnea; hemoptysis; bronchial cough; cyanosis; pulmonary edema
- *Fatigue:* present; increased with decreased exercise tolerance
- *Irregular heartbeat:* usually absent
- *Peripheral changes:* extremity pain; peripheral edema
- *Abdominal pain:* present

History
- Most common in women under age 45
- Recent bronchitis or upper respiratory tract infection may worsen symptoms.
- Patient's past medical history includes rheumatic fever, congenital valve disorder, or tumor (myxoma).

Physical examination
- Inspection reveals malar flush; in young patients, precordial bulge and diffuse pulsation.
- Palpation reveals tapping sensation over area of expected apical impulse, middiastolic and/or presystolic thrill at apex, small pulse, overactive right ventricle with elevated pulmonary pressure.
- Palpation may reveal enlargement of the liver.
- Palpation may reveal irregular, faint pulse and low blood pressure.
- Auscultation reveals localized, delayed, rumbling, low-pitched diastolic murmur at or near apex (duration of murmur varies depending on severity of stenosis; onset of murmur at opening snap early in diastole); possibly loud S_2 with elevated pulmonary pressure; normal blood pressure.

Diagnostic studies
- Electrocardiogram shows notched and broad P waves in standard leads; inverted P in V_1 lead; atrial fibrillation common.
- X-ray examination and fluoroscopy show left atrial enlargement.
- Echocardiography helps assess severity of stenosis.
- Cardiac catheterization and angiocardiography help determine amount of regurgitation that may also be present.

Continued

Conditions Affecting Valvular Function
Continued

MITRAL REGURGITATION (INCOMPETENCE)

Chief complaints
- *Chest pain:* absent
- *Dyspnea:* present, progressive with exertion; orthopnea, paroxysmal dyspnea; cough
- *Fatigue:* present, progressive with exertion
- *Irregular heartbeat:* present as palpitations
- *Peripheral changes:* none

History
- Past medical history includes rheumatic fever, endocarditis, congenital mitral valve defect, papillary muscle dysfunction or rupture, chordae tendineae dysfunction or rupture, heart failure associated with left ventricular dilation, blunt injury to the chest.
- More common in men than in women.
- Mitral incompetence is less common than mitral stenosis.

Physical examination
- Inspection reveals forceful apical impulse to left of left midclavicular line.
- Palpation reveals forceful, brisk apical impulse; systolic thrill over apical impulse; normal, small, slightly collapsing pulse, or irregular pulse.
- Auscultation reveals blowing, high-pitched, harsh, or musical pansystolic apical murmur maximal at apex and transmitted to axilla; abnormally wide splitting of S_2; possibly S_3 present; normal blood pressure.

Diagnostic studies
- Electrocardiogram shows P waves broad or notched in standard leads; with pulmonary hypertension, tall, peaked P waves, right axis deviation, or right ventricular hypertrophy; possibly atrial fibrillation.
- X-ray examination shows enlargement of left ventricle and moderate aneurysmal dilatation of left atrium.
- Echocardiography shows dilated left ventricle and left atrium; pattern of contraction of left ventricle suggests diastolic overload.
- Cardiac catheterization and ventriculography help determine amount of regurgitation and identify prolapsing cusps.

Continued

Conditions Affecting Valvular Function
Continued

PULMONIC STENOSIS

Chief complaints
● *Chest pain:* usually not present
● *Dyspnea:* present on exertion; cyanosis from abnormally low oxygen saturation in the systemic tissues
● *Fatigue:* present
● *Irregular heartbeat:* absent
● *Peripheral changes:* peripheral edema possible
● Patient may be asymptomatic
History
● Congenital stenosis or rheumatic heart disease, associated with other congenital heart defects, such as tetralogy of Fallot
● Infective endocarditis and, rarely, trauma.
Physical examination
● Inspection reveals jugular vein distention.
● Palpation reveals hepatomegaly.
● Auscultation reveals systolic murmur at left sternal border and split S_2 sound, with delayed or absent pulmonic component.
Diagnostic studies
● Electrocardiogram shows right ventricular hypertrophy, right axis deviation, right atrial hypertrophy.
● Chest X-ray shows decreased pulmonary vascular markings in the presence of pulmonary stenosis.
● Echocardiogram shows right ventricular enlargement.

PULMONIC REGURGITATION (INCOMPETENCE)

Chief complaints
● *Chest pain:* absent
● *Dyspnea:* present; cyanosis from abnormally low oxygen saturation in the systemic tissues
● *Fatigue:* present; patient tires easily; weakness; malaise
● *Irregular heartbeat:* absent
● *Peripheral changes:* peripheral edema
History
● Pulmonary hypertension
● Congenital defect
● Endocarditis
● Trauma
● Rheumatic fever
Physical examination
● Inspection reveals jugular vein distention.
● Palpation reveals hepatomegaly.
● Pulsation can generally be felt at second left intercostal space.
● Auscultation reveals diastolic murmur in pulmonic area. Murmur increases with inspiration.
Diagnostic studies
● Electrocardiogram shows right ventricular or right atrial enlargement and right axis deviation.
● Chest X-ray may reveal right ventricular enlargement.
● Echocardiogram will show enlargement or dilatation of the right ventricle.

Guide to Breath Sounds

This chart tells you four things: what you'll hear when you listen to your patient's breath sounds; where you'll hear them; where you *shouldn't* hear certain breath sounds; and what it indicates if you do.

TYPE/ DESCRIPTION	POSITION IN RESPIRATORY CYCLE	NORMALLY HEARD OVER	ABNORMALLY HEARD OVER
Vesicular High-pitched and loud on inspiration; low-pitched and soft on expiration	More prominent during inspiration than during expiration	Peripheral lung fields	Peripheral lung fields in decreased volume; possibly indicating emphysema or pleural effusion
Bronchial or tracheal High-pitched, loud, harsh, hollow	Less prominent during inspiration than during expiration	Trachea and the anterior of the mainstem bronchi	Peripheral lung fields; possibly indicating consolidation, as in pneumonia
Bronchovesicular Moderate pitch and loudness	Equally prominent during inspiration and expiration	Major bronchi, upper anterior chest and posteriorly between scapulae	Peripheral lung fields; possibly an early indication of respiratory disease

Guide to Adventitious Sounds

TYPE/ DESCRIPTION	POSITION IN RESPIRATORY CYCLE	POSSIBLE CAUSE	POSSIBLE INDICATIONS
Fine crackles High-pitched, crackling, and popping	End of inspiration	Fluid in the smallest airways	Pneumonia or congestive heart failure (CHF)
Coarse crackles Low-pitched and loud	Inspiration and expiration	Fluid in the bronchi and trachea	Severe pulmonary edema
Wheeze High-pitched, musical, and squeaky	Predominant in expiration	Air passing through swollen small airways	Asthma or emphysema
Rhonchi Lower-pitched and moaning	Throughout respiratory cycle; may clear with coughing	Air passing through swollen large airways	Bronchitis, tracheobronchitis
Pleural rub Coarse, grating, and low-pitched	Throughout respiratory cycle	Inflamed surfaces of pleurae rubbing together	Pleurisy, tuberculosis, infection, pneumonia, or cancer

Identifying Respiratory Patterns

TYPE OF RESPIRATION	PATTERN	POSSIBLE CAUSES
Apnea: absence of breathing may be periodic	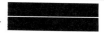	• Airway obstruction • Conditions affecting the brain's respiratory center
Apneustic: prolonged, gasping inspiration, followed by extremely short inefficient expiration	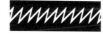	• Lesions of the lateral medulla oblongata
Biot's: fast, deep respirations marked by abrupt pauses. Each breath has the same depth.	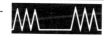	• Spinal meningitis or other central nervous system conditions
Bradypnea: slow, regular respirations	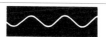	• Conditions affecting the lateral medulla oblongata: tumors, metabolic disorders, decompensation; use of opiates and alcohol • Normal pattern during sleep
Cheyne-Stokes: fast, deep respirations, punctuated by a period of apnea.	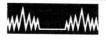	• Increased ICP, severe CHF, renal failure, meningitis, drug overdose, cerebral anoxia

Continued

RESPIRATORY DISORDERS

Identifying Respiratory Patterns
Continued

TYPE OF RESPIRATION	PATTERN	POSSIBLE CAUSES
Eupnea: normal rate and rhythm. Rate varies with age: adult, usually 15 to 17 breaths/minute (bpm); teenagers, usually 12 to 20 bpm; ages 2 to 12, usually 20 to 30 bpm; infants, usually 30 to 50 bpm. Two or three deep breaths normally occur each minute.	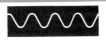	• Normal respiration
Hypernea: deep respirations, normal rate	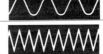	• Strenuous exercise
Kussmaul's: fast (over 20 breaths/minute), deep (resembling sighs), labored respirations without pause		• Renal failure or metabolic acidosis, particularly diabetic ketoacidosis
Tachypnea: rapid respirations. Rate rises with body temperature—about four breaths/minute for every degree Fahrenheit above normal.	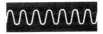	• Fever, as the body tries to rid itself of excess heat • Pneumonia, compensatory respiratory alkalosis, respiratory insufficiency, lesions of the lateral medulla oblongata, and salicylate poisoning

Identifying Percussion Sounds

Use this chart to help you identify the sounds you may hear when you percuss your patient's chest. Be sure to document your findings.

SOUND/ PITCH	INTENSITY	QUALITY	INDICATIONS
Flatness High	Soft	Extreme dullness	*Normal:* sternum; *abnormal:* atelectatic lung
Dullness Medium	Medium	Thudlike	*Normal:* liver area, cardiac area, diaphragm; *abnormal:* pleural effusion
Resonance Low	Moderate to loud	Hollow	*Normal:* lung
Hyper-resonance Lower than resonance	Very loud	Booming	*Abnormal:* emphysematous lung or pneumothorax
Tympany High	Loud	Musical, drumlike	*Normal:* stomach area; *abnormal:* air-distended abdomen

Recognizing the Stages of ARDS

STAGES/SIGNS AND SYMPTOMS	NURSING INTERVENTIONS
Stage 1: Inflamed and damaged alveolocapillary membrane • Depend on underlying cause of ARDS	• Do a brief assessment. • Take the patient's vital signs. • Auscultate for abnormal breath sounds. • Prepare the patient for a chest X-ray. • Begin treatment of underlying cause to prevent further ARDS development.
Stage 2: Protein and water shift in the interstitial space • Tachypnea, dyspnea, and tachycardia	• Draw blood for ABGs. • Prepare the patient for oxygen therapy, intubation, and mechanical ventilation. • Begin fluid management, avoiding fluid overload.
Stage 3: Pulmonary edema • Increased tachypnea, dyspnea, and cyanosis • Hypoxemia (generally unresponsive to increased FIO_2) • Decreased pulmonary compliance • Crackles, wheezes, and rhonchi	• Connect the patient to a mechanical ventilator with a positive end-expiratory pressure (PEEP) setting and a high oxygen concentration. • Watch for complications from ventilator therapy.

Continued

Recognizing the Stages of ARDS
Continued

STAGES/SIGNS AND SYMPTOMS	NURSING INTERVENTIONS
Stage 4: Collapsed alveoli and impaired gas exchange • Thick, frothy, sticky sputum • Marked hypoxemia with increased respiratory distress	• Anticipate that a Swan-Ganz catheter will be inserted to measure pulmonary artery and pulmonary capillary wedge pressure.
Stage 5: Decreased oxygen and carbon dioxide levels in the blood • Increased tachypnea • Hypoxemia • Hypocapnia	• Study ABGs, mixed venous blood gases, and pulmonary capillary wedge pressure to understand the relationship between PEEP, intrapulmonary shunt, and cardiac output. • Monitor the patient's vital signs and urine output (hydration).
Stage 6: Hypoxemia; metabolic acidosis • Decreased serum pH • Increased $Paco_2$ level • Decreased $Paco_2$ level • Decreased HCO_3 level • Confusion	• Watch for hypovolemia, hypotension, and hypoperfusion that may result from fluid restriction or overdiuresis. • Check for shock, coma, respiratory failure, and neurologic complications secondary to metabolic alterations and respiratory failure. • Reassure the patient and his family.

Acid-Base Disorders

Arterial blood gas (ABG) analysis evaluates gas exchange in the lungs by measuring the partial pressures of oxygen (PaO_2) and carbon dioxide ($PaCO_2$) and the pH of an arterial blood sample. PaO_2 indicates how much oxygen the lungs are delivering to the blood. $PaCO_2$ indicates how efficiently the lungs eliminate carbon dioxide. The pH indicates the acid-base measurement of the blood, or the hydrogen ion (H^+) concentration. Acidity indicates H^+ excess; alkalinity, H^+ deficit. Oxygen content (O_2CT), oxygen saturation (O_2Sat), and bicarbonate (HCO_3^-) values also aid diagnosis. A blood sample for ABG analysis may be drawn by percutaneous arterial puncture or from an arterial line.

DISORDERS AND ABG FINDINGS	POSSIBLE CAUSES	SIGNS AND SYMPTOMS
Respiratory acidosis (excess CO_2 retention) pH < 7.35 HCO_3^- > 26 mEq/liter (if compensating) $PaCO_2$ > 45 mm Hg	• CNS depression from drugs, injury, or disease • Asphyxia • Hypoventilation due to pulmonary, cardiac, musculoskeletal, or neuromuscular disease	• Diaphoresis, headache, tachycardia, confusion, restlessness, apprehension
Respiratory alkalosis (excess CO_2 excretion) pH > 7.42 HCO_3^- < 22 mEq/liter (if compensating) $PaCO_2$ < 35 mm Hg	• Hyperventilation due to anxiety, pain, or improper ventilator settings • Respiratory stimulation by drugs, disease, hypoxia, fever, or high room temperature • Gram-negative bacteremia	• Rapid, deep respirations; paresthesias; lightheadedness; twitching; anxiety; fear

Continued

Acid-Base Disorders
Continued

DISORDERS AND ABG FINDINGS	POSSIBLE CAUSES	SIGNS AND SYMPTOMS
Metabolic acidosis (HCO_3^- loss, acid retention) pH < 7.35 HCO_3^- < 22 mEq/liter $PaCO_2$ < 35 mm Hg (if compensating)	• HCO_3^- depletion due to renal disease, diarrhea, or small bowel fistulas • Excessive production of organic acids due to hepatic disease; endocrine disorders, including diabetes mellitus; hypoxia; shock; or drug intoxication • Inadequate excretion of acids	• Rapid, deep breathing; fatigue; headache; lethargy; drowsiness; nausea; vomiting; coma (if severe)
Metabolic alkalosis (HCO_3^- retention, acid loss) pH > 7.42 HCO_3^- > 26 mEq/liter $PaCO_2$ > 45 mm Hg (if compensating)	• Loss of hydrochloric acid from prolonged vomiting, gastric suctioning • Loss of potassium due to increased renal excretion, steroid overdose • Excessive alkali ingestion	• Slow, shallow breathing; hypertonic muscles; restlessness; twitching; confusion; irritability; apathy; tetany; seizures; coma (if severe)

Guide to Acute Respiratory Disorders

CROUP

Severe inflammation and obstruction of the upper airway; may be mistaken for and usually follows upper respiratory tract infection; more common in children. Three types exist: acute laryngotracheobronchitis, laryngitis, and acute spasmodic laryngitis. Laryngotracheobronchitis is the most common type of croup.

Causes
• Viral (parainfluenza, influenza, and measles viruses)
• Bacterial (pertussis and diphtheria)

Signs and symptoms
• Inspiratory stridor
• Hoarse or muffled sounds
• Sharp, barklike cough
• Inflammatory edema and possibly spasm, which may obstruct airway and compromise ventilation

For laryngotracheobronchitis:
• Fever
• Edema of the bronchi and bronchioles
• Scattered crackles

For laryngitis:
• Sore throat and cough, possibly progressing to marked hoarseness

For acute spasmodic laryngitis:
• Mild-to-moderate hoarseness and nasal discharge, followed by cough and noisy inspiration
• Labored breathing with rapid pulse and clammy skin

• Suprasternal and intercostal retractions, dyspnea, diminished breath sounds, restlessness

Nursing interventions
• Promote bed rest.
• Administer aspirin or acetaminophen in recommended dosages.
• Obtain throat specimen for culture.
• Urge use of cool-mist humidifier during sleep.
• Instruct parents to monitor cough and breath sounds, hoarseness, cyanosis, respiratory rate and character, restlessness, and fever.
• To relieve a croup spell, tell the parents to carry the child into the bathroom, shut the door, and turn on the hot water.
• To help control coughing, encourage parents to position two or three pillows under the child's head.
• To relieve the child's sore throat, have parents provide water-based ices, such as fruit sherbert and Popsicles. Tell parents to avoid giving milk-based fluids if child is expectorating thick mucus or has difficulty swallowing.
• Warn parents that ear infection and pneumonia are complications of croup that may appear within 5 days after recovery. Tell them to watch for and report the following signs and symptoms immediately: earache, productive cough, high fever, or increased shortness of breath.

Continued

Guide to Acute Respiratory Disorders
Continued

BRONCHITIS

Inflammation of the tracheobronchial tree, more common in adults, especially those with chronic lung disease.

Causes
• Usually viral; secondary bacterial infections are common

Signs and symptoms
• Cough; may or may not be productive
• Coarse rhonchi or wheezes on lung auscultation
• Nasal discharge
• Fever
• Malaise

Nursing interventions
• Promote bed rest for the patient.
• Administer aspirin or acetaminophen in recommended dosages.
• Urge patient to take all the antibiotic medicine prescribed by the doctor, if appropriate.
• Recommend use of cool-mist vaporizer to help loosen secretions.
• Tell patient to use cough medicine with an expectorant to remove secretions.
• Administer oxygen at 2 liters/minute for acute bronchitis to alleviate ventilation problems.
• To aid with pulmonary hygiene, chest physiotherapy—specifically percussion and postural drainage—is performed.
• Hydrate the patient to help remove mucous plugs and counteract dehydration.

INFLUENZA

Acute, highly contagious respiratory tract infection; occurs sporadically or in epidemics, especially during winter.

Cause
• Viral

Signs and symptoms
• Fever
• Malaise
• Myalgia
• Headache
• Sore throat
• Sudden onset of chills
• Cough

Nursing interventions
• Promote bed rest for the patient.
• Suggest increased fluid intake.
• Administer aspirin or acetaminophen in recommended dosages.
• Administer cough medicine with an expectorant to enhance expectoration of secretions.
• If signs and symptoms persist, instruct patient to return to the doctor for further evaluation. He may develop secondary complications, such as pneumonia.

Continued

Guide to Acute Respiratory Disorders
Continued

PHARYNGITIS

Acute or chronic inflammation of the pharynx; may precede naso-pharyngitis; usually lasts 3 to 10 days; most common throat disorder; often occurs in adults who live or work in dusty or dry environments, habitually use tobacco or alcohol, or suffer from chronic sinusitis, persistent coughs, or allergies.

Causes
• Viral
• Bacterial (usually streptococcus)

Signs and symptoms
• Sore throat
• Difficulty swallowing
• Sensation of lump in throat
• Constant urge to swallow
• On physical exam, posterior wall of pharynx appears red and edematous; mucous membranes studded with white or yellow follicles
• Exudate, usually confined to lymphoid areas
• May be accompanied by mild fever, headache, and muscle and joint pain (especially if bacteria's the cause)

Nursing interventions
• Obtain throat specimen for culture to identify causative organism.
• Promote bed rest for the patient.
• Administer aspirin or acetaminophen in recommended dosages.
• Teach patient with chronic pharyngitis how to minimize throat irritation; for example, by using a humidifier while sleeping.
• Tell your patient to gargle with warm salt water to relieve sore throat pain.
• Administer throat lozenges containing a mild anesthetic to relieve sore throat pain.
• Encourage increased fluid intake.
• Watch for signs of dehydration (cracked lips, dry mucous membranes, low urinary output).
• Provide meticulous mouth care to prevent dry lips and oral pyoderma.
• Administer penicillin, as ordered (if bacteria's the cause).
• Refer patient to a self-help group to stop smoking.

Continued

Guide to Acute Respiratory Disorders
Continued

TONSILLITIS

Inflammation of the tonsils; may be acute or chronic; acute form usually lasts 4 to 6 days and commonly affects children between ages 5 and 10.

Causes
- Bacterial (usually beta-hemolytic streptococcus)
- Viral

Signs and symptoms
For acute tonsillitis:
- Mild-to-severe sore throat
- Loss of appetite (in young child)
- Dysphagia
- Fever
- Chills
- Swelling and tenderness of lymph glands in submandibular area
- Muscle and joint pain
- Malaise
- Headache
- Possibly earache
- Generalized inflammation of pharyngeal wall
- Possibly edematous and inflamed uvula
- Swollen tonsils with white or yellow exudate

For chronic tonsillitis:
- Recurrent sore throat
- Purulent drainage in tonsillar crypts
- Frequent attacks of acute tonsillitis
- Peritonsillar abscess

Nursing interventions
- Administer aspirin or acetaminophen in recommended dosages.
- Administer antibiotics, as ordered (if bacteria's the cause).
- Obtain throat specimen for culture to determine infecting organism and appropriate antibiotic therapy (if bacteria's the cause).
- Use differential diagnosis to rule out infectious mononucleosis and diphtheria.
- Suggest gargling to soothe the throat, unless it exacerbates the pain.
- Make sure the patient and parents understand the importance of completing prescribed course of antibiotic therapy.
- Encourage increased fluid intake.
- Promote bed rest.
- Suggest that parents give child ice cream or flavored drinks and ices.
- If tonsil removal is necessary, explain the procedure.

Continued

RESPIRATORY DISORDERS

Guide to Acute Respiratory Disorders
Continued

ACUTE BACTERIAL SINUSITIS

Inflammation of the paranasal sinus mucosa; recurrence may lead to chronic condition.
Causes
● Bacterial (pneumococcus)
● Viral *(Hemophilus influenzae)*
● Allergy
Signs and symptoms
● Nasal congestion, followed by gradual buildup of pressure in the affected sinus; difficulty in breathing through the nose
● Possibly purulent nasal discharge
● Low-grade fever
● Sore throat
● Malaise
● Nausea and anorexia
● Pain and swelling over the affected sinus
● Periorbital edema
Nursing interventions
● Stress to your patient the importance of taking the antibiotic medication ordered by the doctor.
● Advise your patient to take an oral antihistamine-decongestant combined with aspirin or acetaminophen.
● Teach your patient how to use nasal decongestant spray correctly.
● Encourage fluid intake to mobilize secretions and promote drainage.
● Tell your patient to watch for and report any of the following signs and symptoms of complications: vomiting, chills, fever, edema of forehead or eyelids, blurred or double vision, or personality changes.

NASOPHARYNGITIS

Infection causing mucosal edema and vasodilation.
Cause
● Viral (usually rhinovirus)
Signs and symptoms
● Possibly fever, especially in infants and young children
● Dry, irritated nose and throat, possibly accompanied by sneezing and coughing
● Irritability and restlessness
● Chills
● Muscle soreness
● Vomiting or diarrhea possible in infants and young children
Nursing interventions
● Promote bed rest.
● Administer aspirin or acetaminophen in recommended dosages.
● Instruct patient to gargle with warm saline solution to relieve discomfort.
● If ordered, obtain a throat specimen for culture to test for streptococcal infection.
● Encourage increased fluid intake to loosen secretions and promote drainage.
● Teach patient how to use nose drops to relieve nasal congestion.
● Also tell patient to use antihistamine-decongestant tablets to relieve nasal congestion.

Guide to Chronic Lung Diseases

Here are some general guidelines for you to follow when caring for a patient with chronic lung disease:

Alert your patient to factors that may make his condition worse. These may include stress or anxiety; pollution; excess work, eating, or exercise; and fatigue or lack of sleep.

Show the patient how to breathe through pursed lips to help increase his lung capacity. Also demonstrate relaxation techniques.

Demonstrate chest physiotherapy and postural drainage techniques to your patient.

Emphasize the importance of good mouth care to your patient to help reduce the risk of further infection.

If your patient's receiving oxygen therapy, tell him and his family to administer it in low concentrations.

ASTHMA

Increased bronchial reactivity to stimuli, producing episodic bronchospasm and airway obstruction.
Causes
• *Extrinsic asthma:* exposure to specific allergens, such as ragweed.
• *Intrinsic asthma:* respiratory tract infections; smoke, cold air, atmospheric pollutants; exercise, resulting in hypocapnia; overuse of medications, such as narcotics and sedatives, resulting in hypoventilation and bronchoconstriction; emotionally stressful situations, such as fear or excitement, which cause hyperventilation and hypocapnia
Signs and symptoms
• History of intermittent attacks of dyspnea and wheezing
• Audible wheezing
• Chest tightness (patient feels like he can't breathe)
• Productive cough with thick mucus

• Prolonged expiration
• Intercostal and supraclavicular retraction on inspiration
• Nostril flaring
• Use of accessory muscles during breathing
• Increased chest circumference
• Tachypnea
• Tachycardia
• Perspiration
• Flushing
• Possible signs and symptoms of eczema or allergic rhinitis
• Absent or diminished breath sounds during severe obstruction
• Chest X-ray reveals hyperinflated lungs with trapped air during attack; normal chest X-ray when in remission
• Pulmonary function tests during an attack show decreased forced expiratory volumes, which improve after use of bronchodilator; residual volume and, occasionally, total lung capacity may be normal between attacks.

Continued

RESPIRATORY DISORDERS

Guide to Chronic Lung Diseases
Continued

ASTHMA *Continued*

Nursing interventions
• Administer aerosol containing beta-adrenergic agents or oral beta-adrenergic agents, oral methylxanthines, and steroids to produce bronchodilation and facilitate mucus transport.
• Prepare patient to undergo skin test to try to determine specific allergens causing the condition. If specific allergens can be identified, teach the patient how to avoid them.
• Show patient how to use antihistamines, decongestants, and oral or aerosol bronchodilators, if appropriate.
• Explain how stress and anxiety affect asthma, and teach patient ways to avoid undue stress and anxiety.
• Warn patient of asthma's association with exercise (particularly running) and cold air. Tell him to avoid both, if possible.
• If patient requires emergency treatment, administer oxygen, corticosteroids, and bronchodilators, such as intravenous aminophylline, and inhaled agents, such as isoproterenol, following approved protocol.
• Teach patient pulmonary rehabilitation techniques, such as abdominal/diaphragmatic breathing, relaxation techniques, range-of-motion exercises, and chest physiotherapy.

DIFFUSE INTERSTITIAL PULMONARY FIBROSIS

Progressive thickening and scarring of interalveolar septa, with steadily progressive dyspnea; may result in death from lack of oxygen or heart failure.
Cause
• Inhalation of dust, industrial irritants, allergens, irritant gases, or chemicals.
Signs and symptoms
• Chest pain
• Dyspnea on exertion
• Dry, irritating cough, progressing to productive hemoptysis
• Wheezing
• Tachypnea
• Cyanosis on exertion
• If chemicals are the cause: burning of eyes, nose, throat, and trachea; possibly nausea and vomiting.
Nursing interventions
• Tell patient to control dyspnea by limiting his activity.
• After taking patient's history and determining the cause, warn him to avoid contact with cause.

Continued

Guide to Chronic Lung Diseases
Continued

EMPHYSEMA

Abnormal, irreversible enlargement of air spaces distal to terminal bronchioles, from destruction of alveolar walls; results in decreased elastic recoil properties of lungs.

Cause
● Unknown but believed to be related to deficiency of alpha$_1$-antitrypsin; this deficiency allows release of proteolytic enzymes, which destroy lung tissue; loss of lung-supporting structure results in decreased elastic recoil and airway collapse on expiration; obstruction of alveolar walls decreases surface area available for gas exchange; factors that may be involved include cigarette smoking, respiratory tract infections, air pollution, and allergens.
● Insidious onset
● Dyspnea
● Chronic cough
● Anorexia
● Weight loss
● Chronic malaise
● Increased chest circumference (barrel-chest appearance)
● Use of accessory muscles during breathing
● Prolonged expiratory period with grunting
● Pursed-lip breathing
● Tachypnea
● Peripheral cyanosis
● Digital clubbing
● In advanced disease: flattened diaphragm, reduced vascular markings at lung periphery, overaeration of lungs, vertical heart, enlarged anteroposterior chest circumference, and large retrosternal air space may be visible on chest X-ray
● Pulmonary function tests show increased volume, total lung capacity, and compliance; decreased vital capacity, diffusing capacity, and expiratory volume.

Nursing interventions
● Teach your patient to use bronchodilators to reverse bronchospasm and promote mucociliary clearance
● Stress to your patient the importance of taking antibiotics as ordered to prevent a respiratory tract infection; a flu vaccine to prevent influenza; and Pneumovax to prevent pneumococcal pneumonia.
● Promote fluid intake to help loosen secretions.
● Teach patient and his family how to perform postural drainage and chest physiotherapy at home, if ordered.
● Urge patient to stop smoking. If necessary, refer him to a self-help group. Also, have the patient try to avoid contact with air pollutants.

Continued

Guide to Chronic Lung Diseases
Continued

CANCER

Usually develops within the wall or epithelium of the bronchial tree; various types include a squamous cell (epidermoid), oat cell (small cell), adenocarcinoma, and anaplastic (large cell). Lung cancer is the most common form of cancer causing death.

Cause
• Most likely, the inhalation of carcinogenic pollutants; direct relationship between increased incidence of cancer and cigarette smoking; increased susceptibility for persons working in industries using carcinogenic substances or with family history of cancer.

Signs and symptoms
• Usually do not appear until disease's later stages; depends on the type of cancer and how far it's spread
• Esophageal compression causes dysphagia
• Vena caval obstruction can cause venous distention and edema of the face, neck, chest, and back
• Initially, productive cough, possibly containing mucopurulent or blood-tinged sputum

In squamous cell or oat cell:
• Hemoptysis
• Wheezing

• Dyspnea
• Smoker's cough
• Chest pain later in disease

In adenocarcinoma and anaplastic carcinoma:
• Anorexia, weight loss
• Weakness; fatigue
• Lesion visible on chest X-ray

Nursing interventions
• Since surgery, radiation, and chemotherapy are the most common treatments, your care involves identifying people at risk, early detection of disease, teaching the patient about the procedures and helping prepare him for them, and providing emotional support during treatment.
• Explain the possible side effects of radiation or chemotherapy treatments.
• Explain postop procedures, such as insertion of a Foley catheter or endotracheal tube, I.V. therapy, or dressing changes.
• If patient smokes, urge him to quit. Refer him to a self-help group, if necessary.
• Recommend that all heavy smokers over age 40 have chest X-rays and sputum cytologies annually. Tell your patient to contact his doctor if he detects any change in the character of his cough.

Continued

Guide to Chronic Lung Diseases
Continued

CHRONIC BRONCHITIS

Excessive mucus production in the tracheobronchial tree with productive cough for at least 3 months a year for 2 successive years; severity related to amount and duration of smoking; may worsen during respiratory tract infection; does not usually develop into a significant airway obstruction.

Cause
• Hypertrophy and hyperplasia of the mucus-secreting glands of the trachea, bronchi, and bronchioles, resulting in damage to cilia lining the lungs; cilia's function of clearing the lungs is impaired, and mucous plugs form, becoming a culture medium for bacterial infections.

Signs and symptoms
• Insidious onset
• Productive cough (with clear sputum) that worsens in morning
• Dyspnea on exertion
• Abundant sputum production; may be gray, white, or yellow
• Weight gain from edema
• Cyanosis
• Edema
• Tachypnea
• Digital clubbing (in later stages)
• Wheezing
• No use of accessory muscles noted during respirations
• Prolonged expirations

• Crackles and wheezing on auscultation
• Neck vein distention
• Nasopharyngitis associated with increased sputum and worsening dyspnea may take longer to resolve
• Hyperinflation and increased bronchovascular markings may be visible on X-ray
• Pulmonary function tests show increased residual volume, decreased vital capacity and forced expiratory volumes, normal static compliance and diffusing capacity.

Nursing interventions
• Remind patient of the importance of complying with the antibiotic therapy prescribed by the doctor.
• Urge patient to quit smoking. Refer him to a self-help group for assistance.
• Tell patient to avoid air pollutants.
• Encourage fluid intake to promote secretions.
• Teach patient and his family how to perform chest physiotherapy and postural drainage.
• Teach patient abdominal/diaphragmatic breathing and relaxation techniques.
• Instruct patient and family on the proper use of nebulizers and oxygen therapy.

RESPIRATORY DISORDERS

Assessing for Fat Emboli Syndrome

One of the most serious complications of long-bone fractures is fat emboli syndrome (FES), which may occur 24 to 72 hours after the patient's injury. If FES isn't treated quickly, it can cause acute respiratory distress and death. So notify the doctor *immediately* if you detect the development of FES.

Watch your patient for the following signs and symptoms, and be prepared to intervene appropriately.

SIGNS AND SYMPTOMS

• Altered mental status (in early FES stages)

• Complaint of chest pain on inspiration

• Changes in EKG waveforms (due to chemical irritation)—prominent S waves, T-wave inversions, multiple dysrhythmias, right bundle branch block

• Cardiovascular collapse

• Gradually increasing tachypnea and tachycardia, crackles, wheezing

• Arterial blood gas measurements showing respiratory alkalosis, hypoxemia, pulmonary shunt

• Petechiae (lasting 4 to 6 hours) over the patient's torso, in his axillary folds, in his conjunctival sacs, retina, and soft palate mucosa

• Fever due to brain-center irritation

• Localized muscle weakness, spasticity, and rigidity from muscle irritation

NURSING INTERVENTIONS

• Administer fluids to prevent shock and to dilute free fatty acids.

• Administer corticosteroids, as ordered, to counteract the inflammatory response to free fatty acids.

• Administer digoxin, as ordered, to increase the patient's cardiac output.

• Reassure the patient. He may be frightened or anxious from the hypoxemia.

Recognizing Abnormal Postures

A patient exhibiting any of the three abnormal postures described here may have severe neurologic damage. If your patient assumes any of these postures, alert the doctor immediately.

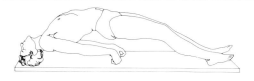

Opisthotonos: characterized by a rigidly arched neck and spine; may indicate meningeal irritation or seizures

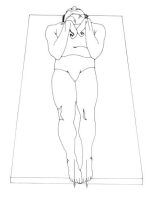

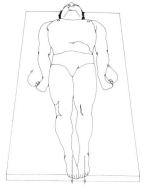

Decorticate posturing: a rigid spine, inwardly flexed arms, extended legs, and plantar flexion; may indicate a lesion at the level of the diencephalon

Decerebrate posturing: a rigid and possibly arched spine, rigidly extended arms and legs, and plantar flexion; may indicate a brain stem lesion

Using the Glasgow Coma Scale

The Glasgow Coma Scale provides a standard reference for assessing or monitoring a patient with suspected or confirmed brain injury. It measures three faculties' responses to stimuli—*eye opening, motor response,* and *verbal response*—and assigns a number to each of the possible responses within these categories. A score of 3 is the lowest and 15 is the highest. A score of 7 or less indicates coma. This scale is commonly used in the emergency department or at the scene of an accident, and for periodic evaluation of the hospitalized patient.

THE GLASGOW COMA SCALE

FACULTY MEASURED	RESPONSE	SCORE
Eye opening	• Spontaneously	4
	• To verbal command	3
	• To pain	2
	• No response	1
Motor response	• To verbal command	6
	• To painful stimuli (apply knuckle to sternum; observe arms).	
	Localizes pain	5
	Flexes and withdraws	4
	Assumes decorticate posture	3
	Assumes decerebrate posture	2
	No response	1
Verbal response (Arouse patient with painful stimuli, if necessary)	• Oriented and converses	5
	• Disoriented and converses	4
	• Uses inappropriate words	3
	• Makes incomprehensible sounds	2
	• No response	1
	Total:	3 to 15

Note: The *decorticate posture* may indicate a lesion of the frontal lobes, internal capsule, or cerebral peduncles. The *decerebrate posture* may indicate lesions of the upper brain system. The *patient's use of inappropriate words* may indicate either receptive or expressive aphasia. *Incomprehensible sounds* indicate expressive aphasia.

Signs of Increased Intracranial Pressure

Intracranial pressure monitoring measures the pressure exerted by brain tissue, blood, and CSF against the skull. Indications for this procedure include head trauma with bleeding or edema, overproduction or insufficient absorption of CSF, cerebral hemorrhage, and space-occupying brain lesions. Such monitoring can detect elevated ICP early, before clinical danger signs develop. Prompt intervention can then help avert or diminish neurologic damage caused by cerebral hypoxia and shifts of brain mass.

- Deteriorating level of consciousness and sensory responses
- Pupillary dilation (especially unilateral): decreased pupillary light reflex; papilledema
- Loss of motor function

- Rising systolic blood pressure
- Widening pulse pressure
- Bradycardia
- Deteriorating respiratory pattern
- Headache
- Vomiting

Results of Increased Intracranial Pressure

Increased intracranial pressure is usually caused by cellular hypoxia or brain shift or distortion.

Cellular hypoxia. If intracranial pressure (ICP) approaches or exceeds the mean systemic arterial pressure, the brain can't become adequately perfused, and the cells become hypoxic. This, as you know, can lead to brain damage or death.

Brain shift or distortion. The only escape route for a swollen brain is through the tentorial notch. Pressure from an expanding mass (blood or tumor) may push structures out of midline. This results in compression of neurons and nerve tracts. As the displaced brain tissues compete with the brain stem for space in the

tentorial notch, the classic signs and symptoms of brain stem compression will appear:

- decreased LOC from impaired reticular-activating system
- change in pupil size and equality and extraocular movements, indicating impairment of the third, fourth, and sixth cranial nerves
- change in motor response (including onset of hemiparesis or decorticate or decerebrate posturing), indicating cortical or midbrain compression of motor tracts
- changes in vital signs and pattern of respirations (which occur late), indicating great pressure on lower brain stem (pons and medulla).

OTHER BODY SYSTEM DISORDERS

Disorders in Transmission of Nerve Impulses

AMYOTROPHIC LATERAL SCLEROSIS
(Lou Gehrig's disease)

Chief complaints
- *Headache/pain:* pain in arms and legs
- *Motor disturbances:* muscle atrophy and weakness, especially in forearms and hands; impaired speech; difficulty chewing, swallowing, and breathing; choking; excessive drooling; urinary frequency, urgency, and difficulty initiating a stream
- *Sensory deviations:* paresthesias
- *Altered level of consciousness:* depression; crying spells and inappropriate laughter caused by bulbar palsy

History
- Onset usually between ages 40 and 70
- Most common in white males
- Precipitating factors include nutritional deficiency, vitamin E deficiency (damaging cell membranes), autoimmune disorder, interference with nucleic acid production, acute viral infections, and physical exhaustion

Physical examination
- Deep tendon reflexes absent; muscle twitches

MYASTHENIA GRAVIS

Chief complaints
- *Motor disturbances:* progressive muscle weakness during activity; respiratory muscles affected during crisis; dysarthria; dysphagia
- *Sensory deviations:* double vision, weak eye muscles

History
- Onset usually between ages 20 and 40
- Most common in females
- Remissions and exacerbations common
- Symptoms worsen with emotional stress, prolonged exposure to sunlight or cold

Physical examination
- Deep tendon reflexes present
- Double vision, weak eye closure; ptosis; expressionless face; nasal vocal tones; nasal regurgitation of fluids; weak chewing muscles; weak respiratory muscles; weak neck muscles, can't support head; proximal limb weakness (may be asymmetrical)

Continued

Disorders in Transmission of Nerve Impulses
Continued

LANDRY'S OR GUILLAIN-
BARRÉ SYNDROME
(acute idiopathic polyneuritis)

Chief complaints
• *Motor disturbances:* muscle weakness in legs, extending to arms and face in 24 to 72 hours and progressing to total paralysis and respiratory failure; flaccid quadriplegia possible; cranial nerve paralysis; ocular paralysis in about 25% of cases
• *Sensory deviations:* paresthesias, vanishing before muscle weakness occurs
History
• Onset at any age
• Predisposing factors include recent viral or bacterial infection, surgery, influenza vaccination, Hodgkin's disease, lupus erythematosus, gastroenteritis
• Rapid onset of muscular symptoms
Physical examination
• Retinal hemorrhage, sinus tachycardia or bradycardia, choked disk, hypertension, signs of ICP, elevated CSF pressure, cranial nerve (VII) paralysis, symmetrical loss of tendon reflexes, ascending peripheral nerve paralysis or weakness, impaired proprioception, loss of bowel and bladder control, muscle tenderness

MULTIPLE SCLEROSIS
(disseminated sclerosis)

Chief complaints
• *Motor disturbances:* slurred speech, intention tremor, nystagmus (Charcot's triad), spastic paralysis, poor coordination, loss of proprioception, ataxia, transient muscle weakness, incontinence or retention
• *Sensory deviations:* numbness and tingling, vision impairment
• *Altered level of consciousness:* euphoria, emotional instability
History
• Most common in young white adults
• Higher incidence in northern climate
• Genetic tendencies
• Initial attack and subsequent relapses may follow acute infections, trauma, vaccination, serum injections, pregnancy, stress
Physical examination
• Pale optic disk on temporal side, increased deep tendon reflexes, joint contractures and deformities, scanning speech, cranial nerve involvement (vertigo, trigeminal neuralgia), decreased or diminished abdominal reflexes, unsteady gait

Continued

Disorders in Transmission of Nerve Impulses
Continued

GRAND MAL SEIZURE
(generalized, tonic-clonic)

Chief complaints
• *Headache:* present on awakening, possibly accompanied by nausea
• *Motor disturbances:* generalized tonic and clonic movements; residual hemiparesis or monoparesis possible
• *Seizures:* generalized
• *Sensory deviations:* weakness, dizziness, numbness, peculiar sensation
• *Altered level of consciousness:* loss of consciousness; mental confusion after awakening, lasting several hours or days

History
• Onset early in life with idiopathic disorder; can occur at any age with secondary disorders, but those associated with fever commonly occur in children.
• Predisposing factors include, with idiopathic seizure disorders (epilepsy), familial history of seizures, genetic involvement; with secondary seizure disorders, cerebral palsy, birth injury, infectious diseases, meningitis, encephalitis, cerebral trauma, metabolic disturbances, cerebral edema, carbon monoxide poisoning, insulin shock, anoxia, brain tumor, drug overdose, child abuse, noncompliance with medication regimen

Physical examination
• Shrill cry, pupillary change, loss of consciousness, tonic and clonic movements, tongue biting, abnormal respiratory pattern (absent during tonic phase), urinary or fecal incontinence, upward deviation of eyes, excessive salivation

SYRINGOMYELIA

Chief complaints
• *Headache/pain:* painful shoulder
• *Motor disturbances:* weakness; hyporeflexia, hyperreflexia, or areflexia; wasting of muscles at level of spinal cord involvement (usually hands and arms); spasticity of lower levels; nystagmus; atrophy and fibrillation of the tongue
• *Sensory deviations:* anesthesia in hands or face

History
• Onset usually between ages 30 and 50
• Symptoms include spontaneous fractures, painless injuries, ulcers from sensory loss; progress irregular (may be in remission for long period)

Physical examination
• Horner's syndrome, nystagmus, knee or shoulder joint deformities, clonus, spasticity, hyperreflexia
• Loss of deep tendon reflex, gradual loss of pain and temperature sense *Continued*

Disorders in Transmission of Nerve Impulses
Continued

JACKSONIAN SEIZURE
(partial motor and partial sensory)

Chief complaints
- *Motor disturbances:* focal seizures, lesions of motor cortex or strip (jacksonian motor seizure)
- *Seizures:* partial, with no loss of consciousness
- *Sensory deviations:* numbness, tingling of one arm or leg or one half of body, auditory alterations, lesions of the sensory strip (jacksonian sensory seizure)

History
- Predisposing factors include birth injury, trauma, infection, and vascular lesions.

Physical examination
- Clonic twitching begins in one part of body, usually one side of the face or the fingers of one hand, and often progresses from face to hand, to arm, to trunk, to legs on the same side of the body (jacksonian march); if twitching begins in the foot, it may progress reversely through the body; rhythmic clonic movements may affect one area (face, arm, leg) without marching.
- Speech loss possible
- Sensory deviations may also progress.
- May progress to a secondary generalized seizure (grand mal)

POLYNEURITIS

Chief complaints
- *Motor disturbances:* leg weakness or paralysis progressing to arms and trunk; weakness most severe in distal extremities and in extensors; footdrop; ataxia; absent leg reflexes; impairment of bowel and bladder function and sphincter control
- *Sensory deviations:* paresthesias in hands or feet; anesthesia or hyperesthesia in distal parts of arms and legs; impaired vibratory and kinesthetic sensibilities; nerves sensitive to pressure

History
- Precipitating factors include alcohol abuse, inadequate diet and malnutrition, pregnancy, gastrointestinal disorders, vitamin B deficiency, weight loss.
- Common in diabetics over age 50

Physical examination
- Dry, scaly skin on back of wrists and hands, hyperpigmentation of skin, plantar responses absent, abdominal skin reflexes decreased or absent, increased pulse rate possible; reduced or absent patellar and Achilles tendon reflex
- Feet tender in diabetics

Continued

OTHER BODY SYSTEM DISORDERS

Disorders in Transmission of Nerve Impulses
Continued

PSYCHOMOTOR SEIZURE
(focal)

Chief complaints
• *Motor disturbances:* speech disturbance; destructive, aggressive behavior
• *Seizures:* temporal lobe dysfunction (behavior disturbance)
• *Sensory deviations:* olfactory hallucinations and other sensory manifestations, depending on location of focus; feeling of déjà vu and déjà pensé
• *Altered level of consciousness:* slower thought processes, altered consciousness, partial amnesia
History
• Secondary to birth injury or congenital abnormalities in infants, to lesions or trauma in children and adults, to arteriosclerosis in adults
Physical examination
• May begin with aura
• Aura may occur in the form of a hallucination or perceptual illusion
• Characterized by automatisms (patterned behavior): lip smacking, head turning, dressing, undressing
• Extreme psychotic behavior possible

EXTRAMEDULLARY SPINAL TUMORS
(neurinomas, meningiomas, sarcomas)

Chief complaints
• *Headache/pain:* dull aching and soreness of muscles, mild pain along nerve root
• *Motor disturbances:* spastic weakness of muscles below lesion; with severe compression, loss of bladder and bowel control; atrophy of muscles; paraplegia
• *Sensory deviations:* paresthesias; impairment of proprioception and cutaneous sensation below lesion; with severe compression, loss of sensation below lesion
History
• Most common in young and middle-aged adults
• Predisposing factors include Hodgkin's disease and metastatic carcinoma.
• Symptoms worsened by exertion
Physical examination
• Muscle atrophy and impairment of reflexes, depending on location and extent of injury and amount of time since injury occurred; sensory sparing in some cases; with half the cord compressed, Brown-Séquard syndrome

Continued

Disorders in Transmission of Nerve Impulses
Continued

INTRAMEDULLARY SPINAL
TUMOR
(gliomas)

Chief complaints
• *Headache/pain:* sharp, tearing, or boring pain, depending on location of tumor; increased by movement and relieved by change of posture
• *Motor disturbances:* weakness in one or both legs, clumsiness, shuffling or spastic gait, incontinence
• *Sensory deviations:* paresthesias occur after pain diminishes; complete sparing of sensation in legs possible
History
• Possible limb heaviness or feeling as though walking on air
• Symptoms worsened by exertion
Physical examination
• Hyperactive leg reflexes, leg weakness, sensory sparing

INTRACRANIAL TUMORS
(medulloblastomas, meningiomas, astrocytomas, acoustic neuromas, oligodendrogliomas)

Chief complaints
• *Headache/pain:* headache, worse in morning; vomiting
• *Motor disturbances:* motor deficits
• *Seizures:* generalized or focal, depending on site of tumor

• *Sensory deviations:* dependent on which cranial nerve is affected by tumor pressure
• *Altered level of consciousness:* progressive deterioration of intellect; behavior changes possible; decreased level of consciousness with increased intracranial pressure
History
• Medulloblastoma most common in young children
• Meningioma most common in women over age 50
• History of present illness includes progressive deterioration of motor function, increasing frequency and duration of headaches, personality changes
Physical examination
• Signs of increased intracranial pressure: widening pulse pressure and bounding pulse (Cushing's phenomenon), ipsilateral (same side as lesion) pupil dilation and contralateral (opposite side of lesion) muscle weakness (syndrome of Weber), decreasing level of consciousness, irregular respiratory patterns progressing to respiratory arrest, temperature fluctuation, papilledema, decorticate or decerebrate posturing
• Motor and sensory deficits appropriate to affected area

Infection and Injury

MENINGITIS

Chief complaints
● *Headache:* present, with nausea and vomiting
● *Motor disturbances:* exaggerated, symmetrical deep tendon reflexes
● *Seizures:* may occur; generalized
● *Sensory deviations:* visual disturbances, such as photophobia
● *Altered level of consciousness:* irritability, confusion, stupor, or coma

History
● Predisposing factors include otitis media, mastoiditis, ruptured brain abscess, sinus infection, hepatitis, tonsillitis, herpes zoster or herpes simplex, bone or skin infection, heart valve or lung infection, skull fracture, recent surgery to head or face, recent viral or bacterial infection.

Physical examination
● High- or low-grade fever, rash, sinus arrhythmias, photophobia, nuchal rigidity, opisthotonos, back pain, shock, signs of increased intracranial pressure, positive Brudzinski's and Kernig's signs

BRAIN ABSCESS

Chief complaints
● *Headache:* present, with nausea and vomiting
● *Motor disturbances:* hemiplegia, speech disturbances, cranial nerve palsies
● *Seizures:* focal or generalized
● *Sensory deviations:* visual field defect (hemianopia), and others depending on position of abscess
● *Altered level of consciousness:* behavioral changes or loss of consciousness

History
● Predisposing factors include mastoid and nasal sinus disease; bacterial endocarditis; pulmonary, skin, and abdominal infections; head trauma.

Physical examination
● Normal or decreased temperature, papilledema, signs of increased intracranial pressure
● Signs similar to those of meningitis, such as nuchal rigidity, positive Brudzinski's and Kernig's signs.

Continued

Infection and Injury
Continued

ENCEPHALITIS

Chief complaints
• *Headache:* present
• *Motor disturbances:* residual parkinsonian paralysis with acute attack; paralysis; ataxia
• *Seizures:* may occur during acute attack; residual seizures in about 60% of cases
• *Altered level of consciousness:* lethargy or restlessness progressing to stupor and coma; may remain comatose several days, weeks, or longer after acute phase subsides; personality changes; mental deterioration in about 60% of cases

History
• Predisposing factors include mosquito bite, measles, chicken pox, mumps, herpes virus, polio vaccine or virus, syphilis (10 to 25 years after infection).

Physical examination
• Fever, nuchal rigidity, back pain, abnormal EEG, signs of increased intracranial pressure
• With history of syphilis, tremors, dysarthria, generalized convulsions, increased deep tendon reflexes, bilateral Babinski's sign; with history of herpes simplex, progressive confusion, recent memory loss, temporal lobe seizures, increased antibody levels to herpes simplex virus; with history of measles virus, memory impairment, seizures, myoclonic jerks, ataxia

HEAD INJURY

Chief complaints
• *Headache:* varies in intensity and duration; generalized, with nausea and vomiting
• *Motor disturbances:* specific to area of injury; dysphagia; dysarthria; paralysis; ataxia
• *Sensory deviation:* vertigo, tinnitus worsened by change in posture
• *Altered level of consciousness:* unconsciousness varies in depth and duration, depending on severity and area of injury

History
• Some type of fall or accident, such as a vehicular or industrial accident; blow to the head

Physical examination
• Signs of increased ICP, retrograde and posttraumatic amnesia, hyperthermia, shock, scalp bleeding, evidence of other injuries

Disorders Affecting Blood or Cerebrospinal Fluid Circulation

TRANSIENT ISCHEMIC ATTACK

Chief complaints
• *Motor disturbances:* depend on location of affected artery ataxia; dizziness; falling; weakness
• *Sensory deviations:* numbness, depending on location of affected artery; paresthesias; double vision; fleeting monocular blindness
• *Altered level of consciousness:* drowsiness, giddiness, decreased level of consciousness

History
• Higher incidence in black men over age 50
• Symptoms include transient neurologic deficit lasting seconds to no more than 24 hours; hypertension

Physical examination
• Normal neurologic examination between episodes

CEREBROVASCULAR ACCIDENT

Chief complaints
• *Headache/pain:* present, when affecting carotid artery
• *Motor disturbances:* aphasia, dysphasia, contralateral hemiparesis or hemiplegia, weakness, contralateral paralysis or paresis, diplopia, poor coordination, dysphagia, ataxia, impaired motor function, incontinence
• *Sensory deviations:* numbness, tingling, dizziness, deafness, impaired vision, pain and temperature impairment
• *Altered level of consciousness:* mental confusion, poor memory, amnesia, loss of consciousness, personality changes

History
• Precipitating factors include atrial fibrillation, subacute bacterial endocarditis, recent heart valve surgery, lung abscess, tuberculosis, air embolism during abortion, pulmonary trauma, surgery, thrombophlebitis, transient ischemic attack, diabetes mellitus, gout, arteriosclerosis, intracerebral tumors, trauma

Physical examination
• Labored breathing; rapid pulse rate; fever; nuchal rigidity; evidence of emboli to arms, legs, and intestines and other organs, such as spleen, kidneys, or lungs
• When affecting carotid artery, bruits over artery

Continued

Disorders Affecting Blood or Cerebrospinal Fluid Circulation
Continued

ARTERIOVENOUS (AV) MALFORMATION

Chief complaints
• *Headache:* migraine on side of malformation; accompanied by vomiting
• *Motor disturbances:* signs of increased intracranial pressure, depending on area of malformation; paresis and cerebrovascular accident from rupture
• *Seizures:* general, focal, or jacksonian; may be first sign of rupture and result from ischemia
• *Sensory deviations:* visual disturbances; sensory loss, depending on area involved; symptoms same as hemorrhage from cerebrovascular accident
• *Altered level of consciousness:* dementia from brief ischemia
History
• Patient may complain of swishing sensation in head; sudden "stroke" in young patients
Physical examination
• Pulsating exophthalmos from ocular pressure; papilledema; retinal hemorrhage if carotid artery bleeds into cavernous sinus; hydrocephalus if membrane causes pressure on aqueduct of Sylvius; bruits over lesion, which disappear with pressure over ipsilateral carotid artery

CEREBRAL ANEURYSM AND INTRACEREBRAL OR SUBARACHNOID HEMORRHAGE

Chief complaints
• *Headache:* sudden, severe headache, with nausea and projectile vomiting
• *Motor disturbances:* depends on site of aneurysm and degree of bleeding or ischemia; hemiparesis, aphasia, ataxia, vertigo, syncope, facial weakness
• *Seizures:* focal or generalized
• *Sensory deviations:* visual impairment with pressure on optic nerve or chiasm; double vision with third, fourth, and fifth cranial nerve compression
• *Altered level of consciousness:* stupor to coma, irritability
History
• No symptoms until bleeding or rupture
• Hypertension, oral contraceptives, AV malformations, family history, recurrent headaches
Physical examination
• Temperature may reach 102° F. (38.9° C.) or higher; irregular respirations, dilated and fixed pupils, papilledema, retinal hemorrhage, bilateral Babinski's reflex, positive Brudzinski's and Kernig's signs, nuchal rigidity, signs of increased ICP, blood in CSF

Continued

Disorders Affecting Blood or Cerebrospinal Fluid Circulation
Continued

EPIDURAL (acute) AND SUB-DURAL (acute and chronic) HE-MATOMAS

Chief complaints
• *Motor disturbances:* hemiplegia, hemiparesis or facial weakness on opposite side as hematoma
• *Seizures:* generalized
• *Altered level of consciousness:* irritability, mental confusion, and progressively decreasing level of consciousness; with chronic form, severe impairment of intellectual faculties

History
• Signs occur when hematoma has grown large enough to compromise circulation to the brain (increased intracranial pressure).
• With acute form, complaints rapidly develop (within 48 hours).
• With chronic form, complaints develop more slowly (within a few days to weeks).
• Not all lesions (especially chronic) cause signs of increased intracranial pressure.

Physical examination
• Positive Babinski's reflex
• Signs of increased intracranial pressure
• Epidural hematomas cause a rapid rise in intracranial pressure and should be treated as a surgical emergency.

MIGRAINE
(common, hemiplegic, ophthalmo-plegic, basilar artery, temporal artery)

Chief complaints
• *Headache/pain:* with common migraine, recurrent and severe incapacitating headache (unilateral or bilateral), aura with gastric pain; with hemiplegic or ophthalmoplegic migraine, severe unilateral headache; with basilar artery migraine, severe occipital throbbing headache with vomiting; with temporal artery migraine, throbbing unilateral headache, generalized muscle pain
• *Motor disturbances:* with hemiplegic and ophthalmoplegic migraine, extraocular muscle palsy, ptosis, possible permanent third nerve paralysis, hemiplegia; with basilar artery migraine, ataxia, dysarthria
• *Sensory deviations:* with common migraine, aura may include visual flashing lights, hemianopsia, visual field defects, numbness, nausea, vomiting, vertigo, sensitivity to light and noise; with hemiplegic and ophthalmoplegic migraine, hemiparesis; with basilar artery migraine, partial vision loss, vertigo, tinnitus, tingling of fingers and toes; with temporal artery migraine, visual loss

Continued

Disorders Affecting Blood or Cerebrospinal Fluid Circulation
Continued

MIGRAINE
Continued

- *Altered level of consciousness:* with common migraine, aura includes fatigue, depression, anxiety, and euphoria; with temporal artery migraine, confusion, disorientation

History
- Most common in females
- Family history of *sick headache*
- Onset usually around age 30
- Predisposing factors include emotional disturbance, fatigue, or anxiety; intense concentration; oral contraceptives; menstruation; change in routine; hypothyroidism or hyperthyroidism; food additives; drinking wine or sleeping late.
- Temporal artery migraine affects mostly females over age 60

Physical examination
- With common migraine, tearing, pallor or flushing, perspiration, tachycardia during attack, transitory motor or sensory defects, tenderness and prominent blood vessels on head
- With hemiplegic or ophthalmoplegic migraine, ptosis, third cranial nerve dysfunction, hemiplegia
- With basilar artery migraine, ataxia
- With temporal artery migraine, occasional fever; swollen and tender temporal arteries

CLUSTER HEADACHE

Chief complaints
- *Headache/pain:* intense, stabbing eye pain; sudden onset
- *Motor disturbances:* ptosis

History
- More common in men
- Onset same time each day, duration 10 minutes to 2 hours
- Persists from several weeks to several months, then goes into remission for a long period of time
- Triggered by alcohol
- Aggravated by use of vasodilators, such as nitroglycerin or isosorbide dinitrate
- Associated with emotional stress

Physical examination
- Tearing of affected eye
- Red, runny nose
- Sweating on affected side of face
- Horner's syndrome

Guide to Pediatric Developmental Neurologic Disorders

SYDENHAM'S CHOREA
(St. Vitus' dance)

Chief complaints
• *Motor disturbances:* sporadic movements of face, trunk, and extremity muscles; incoordination; muscle weakness; facial grimacing; arthritis; arthralgia (growing pains)
• *Altered level of consciousness:* restlessness, emotional instability
History
• Onset usually between ages 5 and 15; rheumatic fever
• Symptoms include lack of sleep due to involuntary movements, nightmares; progresses over 2 weeks
Physical examination and diagnostic studies
• Muscle weakness, facial grimacing, no muscle atrophy or contractures

DOWN'S SYNDROME

Chief complaints
• *Motor disturbances:* generalized muscular hypotonicity; structural, facial abnormalities
• *Altered level of consciousness:* impaired mental capacity
History
• Family history of Down's syndrome

• Most common in infants born to mothers over age 35 or in first-born of very young mothers
• Growth and development slower than normal
Physical examination and diagnostic studies
• Guttural cry; small, round head; flat, low-set ears; mongoloid slant to eyes; small mouth with protruding tongue; increased fat pad at nape of neck; short, heavy hands; transverse palmar crease (simian crease); Brushfield's spots (gray-white specks on iris)

HYDROCEPHALUS

Chief complaints
• *Motor disturbances:* spastic movements of arms and legs (more severe in legs), hyperactive tendon reflexes
• *Altered level of consciousness:* apathy, lethargy, irritability
History
• Normal head size at birth, increasingly more rapid growth than normal
Physical examination and diagnostic studies
• Head growth exceeds normal by ½" (1.27 cm) per month; distended scalp veins; full, tense fontanelles; widened cranial sutures;

Continued

Guide to Pediatric Developmental Neurologic Disorders
Continued

HYDROCEPHALUS
Continued

asymmetrical appearance of head; setting-sun sign; inability to hold head up; strabismus; cracked-pot sign on skull percussion; high-pitched cry
● Skull transilluminates

SPINA BIFIDA

Chief complaints
● *Motor disturbances:* weakness, loss of tendon reflexes in legs, gait disturbances, incontinence
● *Sensory deviations:* impaired sensations in legs
History
● May be asymptomatic
● Weakness in legs
Physical examination and diagnostic studies
● Palpable defect; scoliosis; valgus, varus, or caries deformities of feet, usually unilateral

REYE'S SYNDROME

Chief complaints
● *Motor disturbances:* in Stage I, none; in Stage II, hyperactive reflexes; in Stage III, decorticate rigidity; in Stage IV, decerebrate rigidity, large and fixed pupils; in Stage V, loss of deep tendon re-flexes, flaccidity
● *Seizures:* none, until Stage V
● *Altered level of consciousness:* in Stage I, lethargy; in Stage II, coma; in Stage III, deepening coma; in Stage IV and V, deep coma
History
● Acute viral infection
● Prodromal symptoms include malaise, cough, earache, rhinorrhea, sore throat
Physical examination and diagnostic studies
● Vomiting and lethargy (Stage I); hyperventilation, delirium, hyperactive reflexes (Stage II); coma, decorticate rigidity (Stage III); large, fixed pupils, decerebrate rigidity (Stage IV); seizures, loss of deep tendon reflexes, respiratory arrest (Stage V).
● Serum ammonia level above 300 mg/dl, elevated BUN and liver enzyme levels, increased intracranial pressure, prolonged prothrombin time, decreased partial pressure of carbon dioxide ($PaCO_2$).

CEREBRAL PALSY
(spastic, athetoid, and ataxic forms)

Chief complaints
● *Motor disturbances:* in spastic form, hyperactive deep tendon reflexes, rapid alternating muscle contractions and relaxations; in

Continued

OTHER BODY SYSTEM DISORDERS

Guide to Pediatric Developmental Neurologic Disorders
Continued

CEREBRAL PALSY
Continued

athetoid form, grimacing, dystonia, wormlike movements, sharp and jerky movements before becoming more severe during stress and disappearing during sleep; in ataxic form, muscle weakness, loss of balance and coordination, especially in arms
• *Seizures:* in spastic form, seizure disorders possible
• *Sensory deviations:* in spastic form, visual and hearing deficits possible
• *Altered level of consciousness:* in ataxic form, emotional disorders, mental retardation in about 40% of cases
History
• Maternal infection, especially rubella
• Prenatal radiation, anoxia
• Birth difficulties, such as forceps delivery, breech presentation, placenta previa, premature birth
• Infection or trauma during infancy, such as brain infection; head trauma; prolonged anoxia
Physical examination and diagnostic studies
• Underdeveloped affected limbs; hard-to-separate legs; leg crossing, rather than bicycling, when

child's lifted from behind; scissors gait; muscle weakness; hyperactive reflexes; contractures; persistent favoring of one hand; nystagmus; dental abnormalities

NEUROFIBROMATOSIS
(von Recklinghausen's disease)

Chief complaints
• *Headache;* pain along nerve distribution
• *Motor disturbances:* rarely any weakness or atrophy
• *Altered level of consciousness:* may occur with brain tumor
History
• Onset may be any time from childhood to age 50
• Family history of neurofibromatosis—congenital
• May be accompanied by meningiomas, gliomas of the central nervous system
Physical examination and diagnostic studies
• Multiple tumors under the skin of the scalp, arms, legs, trunk, and on cranial nerves; pigmentary lesions, café au lait spots; symptoms similar to brain or spinal tumor, depending on tumor's location; overgrowth of skin and of skull and neck tissue; hypertrophy of face, tongue, arms, and legs; skeletal anomalies; bone cysts

Continued

Guide to Pediatric Developmental Neurologic Disorders
Continued

NEUROFIBROMATOSIS
Continued

• Cranial nerve abnormalities if affected

PETIT MAL SEIZURE
(absence)

Chief complaints
• *Motor disturbances:* myoclonus, automatisms, usually no loss of tone in muscles
• *Seizures:* Petit mal
• *Altered level of consciousness:* brief loss of consciousness characterized by fixed gaze and blank expression; postictal period immediately followed by alertness and continued activity
History
• Idiopathic seizure disorder diagnosed usually between ages 4 and 12; onset rare after age 20
• Predisposing factors include birth injury or developmental de-

fect, acute febrile illness
Physical examination and diagnostic studies
• Petit mal triad: myoclonic jerks, automatisms, transient absences
• May be characterized only by brief staring periods with occasional eye blinks

INFANTILE SPASM

Chief complaint
• *Motor disturbances:* sudden dropping of the head and flexing of the arms; clonic movements of the arms and legs; developmental and mental retardation
History
• Usually lasts until age 4, then possibly changes to generalized seizures
Physical examination and diagnostic studies
• Brief myoclonic jerks involving entire body
• EEG changes

OTHER BODY SYSTEM DISORDERS

Documenting a Seizure

To properly document a seizure, you must collect as much information as you can about the seizure, the child's medical history, and his present physical condition.

Suppose you didn't witness the seizure. Then get an accurate description from someone who did, such as a babysitter, brother, sister, or the parents. Find out what the patient was doing immediately before the seizure and what type of care was given during the seizure. Ask if he's been taking any medication or has any chronic illness or allergies. Record the baseline data you'll get from various diagnostic tests.

Be sure to carefully record specific information. The health-care professionals who later care for your patient will need all the information you can provide.

Immediately after your patient's seizure, record the answers to these questions:

• *Eyes:* Did his eyes deviate to one side, stare, or roll? Did he blink slowly or rapidly? Did his pupils change in size, shape, equality, or reaction to light?

• *Face:* Did his face twitch? If on one side only, which side?

• *Head:* Did his head move backward, forward, right, or left?

• *Mouth:* Were his teeth clenched or open? Was he grimacing or chewing?

• *Tongue:* Did it deviate to one side or roll backward?

• *Respirations:* What was his respiratory rate and quality? Was he cyanotic?

• *Motor activity:* Where did the motor activity begin? What parts of his body were involved? Was there a pattern of progression to the activity? Describe twitching, stiffening, or any other movements.

• *State of consciousness:* Was the patient unconscious? If so, for how long? Could you arouse him? Did he fall? Did he immediately go into a deep sleep after the seizure? How much time elapsed before he became fully alert?

• *Seizure awareness:* Is the patient aware of what happened? Was he upset or confused?

• *Body activities:* Did he experience incontinence, vomiting, or excessive salivation?

• *Onset:* Was the seizure's onset sudden or preceded by an aura? If preceded by an aura, have the patient describe what he experienced; or ask someone who witnessed the seizure to describe the patient's behavior immediately prior to the seizure.

• *Duration:* What time did the seizure begin and end?

• *Frequency and number:* Did he have one seizure or several? If several, how close together did they occur?

Guide to Geriatric Neurologic Disorders

PARKINSON'S DISEASE

Chief complaints
• *Motor disturbances:* tremor; characteristic rhythmic, unilateral pill-rolling movement involves thumb and forefinger; muscle rigidity; akinesia; inability to initiate and perform volitional motor activities; slow, shuffling Parkinson's gait—may be retropulsive or propulsive; fatigue
• *Sensory deviations:* thermal paresthesia, hyperhidrosis, pain in one or both arms
• *Altered level of consciousness:* minor intellectual deficit

History
• Onset usually between ages 50 and 65
• Predisposing factors include family history of parkinsonism; past viral infections, such as influenza
• Symptoms include increasing difficulty performing activities of daily living, slow eating and walking, inability to write in script—reversion to printing
• Increased tremor during stress or anxiety; tremor decreases with purposeful movement and with sleep

Physical examination
• Resistance to passive movement; postural deformities of arms, legs, and trunk; festinating gait; arms fail to swing when walking; cogwheeling; eczema; micrographia; bradykinesia; hand tremor at rest; low, monotone speech pattern

ALZHEIMER'S DISEASE (presenile dementia) and SENILE DEMENTIA

Chief complaints
• *Motor disturbances:* expressive and receptive aphasia, echolalia, apraxia, spatial disorientation, repetitive movements, incontinence
• *Seizures:* possible
• *Altered level of consciousness:* personality changes; progressive dementia; loss of recent memory at first, and then remote memory; decreased attention span; faulty concentration; loss of abstract thinking; restlessness and overactivity

History
• Most common in women over age 50

Physical examination
• Difficulty comprehending written and verbal speech, slow reflexes, shuffling gait, memory changes, hyperactivity, irritability

Postoperative Neurologic Complications

COMPLICATION	LEVEL OF CONSCIOUSNESS	PUPILS
Adverse effects of general anesthesia	• Unconsciousness • Emergence excitement • Hallucinations • Prolonged drowsiness	• Dilated during emergence excitement
Pain	• Alert (if no longer anesthetized) • Anxious	• Dilated, responsive to light
Increased intracranial pressure	• Confusion, progressing to coma	• Unequal
Inappropriate antidiuretic hormone secretion	• Irritability • Decreased level of consciousness	• Dilated
Acute respiratory failure	• Anxious • Depressed • Lethargic • Confused	• Dilated

RESPIRATIONS	MOTOR FUNCTION	OTHER
• Depressed	• Muscle relaxation • Loss of reflexes	• Hypotension • Cardiac dysrhythmias • Temperature alterations • Vomiting
• Rapid	• Restlessness • Increased muscle tension	• Tachycardia • Cool, moist skin
• Slow, dysrhythmic	• Weakened hand grasp, progressing to paralysis, progressing to hyperreflexia, progressing to decerebrate rigidity	• Papilledema • Bradycardia • Hypertension
• Rapid initially, then slow	• Muscle weakness	• Decreased urination, hunger, and thirst
• Increased depth and rate	• Restlessness	• Increased heart rate • Decreased blood pressure • Headache

OTHER BODY SYSTEM DISORDERS

Guide to Common EENT Emergencies

PROBLEM	SIGNS AND SYMPTOMS
Corneal abrasion, corneal ulcer	• Severe eye pain
	• Excessive tearing
	• Reddened conjunctiva
	• Squinting
	• Photophobia
	• History of eye trauma or eye infection
	• Sensation of foreign body in eye
Laceration of the eyeball	• Severe eye pain; poor vision
	• External leakage of ocular fluid
	• Embedded foreign body
	• Blood in anterior chamber of eye
	• History of recent blow to the eye or an injury to surrounding tissue

EMERGENCY NURSING INTERVENTIONS

• If your patient's pain is so severe he can't tolerate an adequate eye examination, administer a topical anesthetic to his affected eye. Be sure to get a doctor's order before you do. Or check your hospital's policy on such things.

• Examine the affected eye with a flashlight. If no lesion's visible but you strongly suspect one, call the doctor. He may instill fluorescein sodium (Ful-Glo Strips*) and examine the eye under a slit lamp or ultraviolet light. Irrigate your patient's eye with artificial tears after the exam.

• If examination reveals a corneal abrasion or ulcer, the doctor may ask you to instill antibiotic ointment and apply an eye patch.

• Apply warm compresses to the affected eye, if ordered, to help relieve discomfort. Be sure your patient's eye is closed *before* you apply a compress to it.

• Give oral medication for pain, if ordered.

• To help relieve photophobia, instruct your patient to wear dark glasses.

• Call the doctor immediately.

• Reassure your patient, and instruct him to lie flat until the doctor arrives. Meanwhile, apply an eye shield to help protect the affected eye. Don't permit the shield to press on the eyeball.

• Get a detailed history of the injury. Include the time of the accident, as well as how it occurred.

• Avoid touching the patient's eye during the examination. Use very *light pressure,* or you'll cause further injury.

• Administer a sedative, as ordered, and prepare your patient for surgery, if his condition requires it.

*Available in the United States and in Canada.

Continued

OTHER BODY SYSTEM DISORDERS

Guide to Common EENT Emergencies
Continued

PROBLEM	SIGNS AND SYMPTOMS
Fractured tooth	• If only the tooth enamel is involved, the fracture site will be rough but not sensitive to touch. • If the dentin is exposed, the tooth may be sensitive to touch or air. The color of the fracture surface will be yellowish brown. • If the fracture has exposed the pulp, the tooth will appear pink. It will be painful when tooth is touched. • If the root is involved, the tooth will be loose. It will be painful when tooth is touched.
Fractured larynx	• Severe face and neck pain • Anterior cervical neck area appears flat • Subcutaneous emphysema over larynx • Nonpalpable thyroid cartilage • Dysphagia and hoarseness
Acute epiglottitis	• Dyspnea or apnea in severe cases • High fever • Inspiratory stridor in children (rarely heard in adults) • Severe sore throat, with cherry-red, enlarged epiglottis • Possible substernal retraction on inspiration • Coughing and hoarseness
Hemorrhage post-tonsillectomy or postadenoidectomy	• Signs of hypovolemic shock: restlessness; agitation; diaphoresis; apprehension; rapid, thready pulse; low blood pressure; and cool, clammy skin • Frank bleeding from mouth

EMERGENCY NURSING INTERVENTIONS

- Gather the following equipment: dental burs, stone or sandpaper disks. The doctor may need these to smooth jagged tooth edges.
- If dentin is involved, cover the fractured area with a clean 2″ x 2″ sterile gauze pad. Administer pain medication, as ordered, while patient waits for the dentist.
- If pulp is exposed, place a sedative dressing on the exposed area, per doctor's order. Prepare for dentist to perform partial pulpotomy or pulpectomy, if necessary.
- If the root is involved, the doctor may want you to give the patient a pain medication. Prepare patient for possible tooth extraction by dentist.

- Don't leave patient.
- Be alert for possible airway obstruction. Have trach set and suction equipment ready.
- Always look for laryngeal trauma or fracture in a patient with multiple injuries. Remember, a halter seat belt can cause fractured larynx in a car accident victim.

- Make sure patient has an open airway. If he's in a seated position, thrust his chest forward and hyperextend his neck.
- Be prepared to assist doctor if he wants to intubate patient or do an emergency tracheotomy.
- Be prepared to start appropriate I.V. therapy with antibiotics and steroids, per doctor's orders.

- After tonsillectomy, depress tongue sufficiently with tongue blade to examine pharynx. Look for blood clot, which may mask posterior bleeding into stomach.
- If patient shows signs of shock, start an I.V. with appropriate solution and draw a blood sample for type and cross matching.
- Gather the following equipment: electrocautery apparatus, sutures, and posterior packs.

*Available in the United States and in Canada.   *Continued*

Guide to Common EENT Emergencies
Continued

PROBLEM	SIGNS AND SYMPTOMS
Contusion of the eyeball	• Eye pain; poor vision • History of recent blow to eye or injury to surrounding tissue (black eye) • Patient complains of blurred vision, spots, or light flashes (all signs of possible retinal detachment)
Perforated eardrum	• Severe ear pain, possibly followed by a sudden decrease in pain as the eardrum ruptures • Ear drainage • Fever • Possible bleeding • Burns in or surrounding ear
Epistaxis	• Frank bleeding from nose • Restlessness; anxiety; apprehension; cool, clammy skin; rapid, thready pulse; low blood pressure (all signs of hypovolemic shock) • Pale mucous membranes in nasal passages • Patient lives or works in hot, unhumidified environment. Has history of nasal injury, recent upper respiratory infection, hypertension, blood dyscrasia, coronary artery disease, or alcoholism.

EMERGENCY NURSING INTERVENTIONS

- Call the doctor immediately.
- *Caution:* During eye examination, don't touch the patient's eye more than once, especially if it feels soft.
- Have patient lie on his back, with his head elevated. Then, cover the affected eye with an eye shield, and apply an ice pack.
- Get a detailed history of the injury.
- If the injury's minor, the doctor may want an ice pack applied to the affected eye for the first 24 hours, then warm compresses every 15 minutes thereafter. Instruct your patient how to apply warm compresses.
- Administer a sedative, as ordered, and prepare your patient for surgery, if his condition requires it.

- Get patient's complete medical history.
- *Caution:* Never irrigate the ear.
- If burns are present, give burn care as needed.
- Give antibiotic ear drops, as ordered.
- Instruct your patient to keep his ear clean and dry. Tell him to place a cotton ball or ear mold inside his outer ear when showering or shampooing.

- Get the patient's medical history. Find out if he's taking any medications for recent illness. Look for Medic Alert bracelet to see if patient has blood dyscrasia.
- If patient has a blood dyscrasia, the doctor may want you to administer vitamin K₁* and plasma.
- Place patient in seated position. Instruct him to pinch his nose shut with 4″ x 4″ sterile gauze pads. Bend his head forward slightly so he won't swallow any blood. If that's unsuccessful, apply ice to back of his neck.
- Have necessary equipment on hand: a nasal speculum; a suction device, with angulated nasal tip; cocaine strips; electrocautery apparatus; silver nitrate sticks; and leads from chromic acid beads.
- If the doctor can't stop the bleeding, he may want you to help insert an anterior or anterior/posterior nasal pack.

*Available in the United States and in Canada.

GI Disorders

GINGIVITIS

Chief complaints
• *Pain:* may be present
• *Nausea/vomiting:* absent
• *Dysphagia:* usually absent
History
• Local irritation, blood dyscrasias, little or no gingival stimulation, mouth breathing, and pregnancy are predisposing factors; most common during puberty.
Physical examination
• Gingival swelling, redness, bleeding, change in normal contour
Diagnostic studies
• None pertinent

APHTHOUS STOMATITIS

Chief complaints
• *Pain:* may be severe
• *Nausea/vomiting:* absent
• *Dysphagia:* may be present
History
• Stress, fatigue, anxiety, and menstruation are predisposing factors; common in young girls.

Physical examination
• Single or multiple shallow ulcers with white centers and red borders
Diagnostic studies
• None pertinent

PERIODONTITIS

Chief complaints
• *Pain:* usually absent at first; later, slightly painful around teeth's supporting area; if abscess develops, severe local pain may occur
• *Nausea/vomiting:* absent
• *Dysphagia:* usually absent
History
• Uncontrolled diabetes, blood dyscrasias, pregnancy, traumatic irritation, and poor oral hygiene are predisposing factors.
• Most common in pubescent females.
Physical examination
• Gingival recession; periodontal pocket containing food, bacteria, calculi; tenderness on palpation; teeth mobility in advanced stage
Diagnostic studies
• Dental X-ray shows destruction of supporting osseous tissues; biopsy provides differential diagnosis.

Continued

GI Disorders
Continued

GLOSSITIS

Chief complaints
- *Pain:* usually present; may be severe
- *Nausea/vomiting:* absent
- *Dysphagia:* usually present

History
- Irritation, injury, poorly fitting or improperly fitted dentures, alcoholism, tobacco smoking, diet of spicy foods, allergy to toothpastes and mouthwashes are predisposing factors; difficulty in speaking and chewing and changes in taste are related signs.

Physical examination
- Reddened, ulcerated, or swollen tongue; swelling may obstruct airway

Diagnostic studies
- None pertinent

HERPES SIMPLEX, PRIMARY (HERPES SIMPLEX TYPE 1 VIRUS)

Chief complaints
- *Pain:* may be severe
- *Nausea/vomiting:* absent
- *Dysphagia:* may be present

History
- Irritability, headache, and fever are related symptoms; most common in children.

Physical examination
- Multiple vesicles that ulcerate rapidly, forming yellow-white ulcers with red halos; lesions may appear on gingival, labial, or buccal mucosa

Diagnostic studies
- Confirmation requires isolation of the virus from local lesions, histologic biopsy, and serologic tests.

ORAL CANCER

Chief complaints
- *Pain:* usually absent; presence depends on location, degree of invasion, and pressure on surrounding tissue
- *Nausea/vomiting:* absent
- *Dysphagia:* usually present only in advanced stages

History
- Smoking or chewing tobacco, overexposure to sunlight, and alcoholism are predisposing factors; most common in men over age 40.

Physical examination
- Early lesions are white with varying texture, or red, soft, and smooth; ulcerating cancer has raised, firm, and fixed margins; may bleed

Diagnostic studies
- Biopsy provides differential diagnosis.

Continued

OTHER BODY SYSTEM DISORDERS

GI Disorders
Continued

NECROTIZING ULCERATIVE GINGIVOSTOMATITIS (VINCENT'S DISEASE, TRENCH MOUTH)

Chief complaints
• *Pain:* may be severe enough to interfere with eating
• *Nausea/vomiting:* absent
• *Dysphagia:* may be severe
History
• Poor oral hygiene, lowered resistance, agranulocytosis, and leukemia are possible predisposing factors; headache and malaise are related symptoms; most common in men ages 20 to 25.
Physical examination
• Ulcerative erosion of gingival papillae, gray pseudomembrane oval covering, low-grade fever, regional lymphadenitis
Diagnostic studies
• Culture may reveal fusiform bacillus or spirochete.

HIATAL HERNIA

Chief complaints
• *Pain:* usually absent; occasional heartburn (gastroesophageal reflux); severe pain if incarcerated
• *Nausea/vomiting:* nocturnal regurgitation, aggravated by lying down, relieved by standing
• *Dysphagia:* if hernia produces esophagitis, esophageal ulceration or stricture

History
• Increased intraabdominal pressure, caused by straining, obesity, ascites, or coughing, is a predisposing factor; most common in elderly women.
Physical examination
• Physical signs absent
Diagnostic studies
• Barium swallow shows pouching in lower esophagus.

ACHALASIA (second-degree abnormal peristalsis or obstructed esophagogastric junction)

Chief complaints
• *Pain:* usually absent
• *Nausea/vomiting:* possible regurgitation of food eaten hours before, without acid taste
• *Dysphagia:* progressive difficulty with both solids and liquids
History
• Weight loss, slowed eating, coughing, wheezing, and choking are related signs and symptoms, aggravated by emotional stress.
Physical examination
• Physical signs absent
Diagnostic studies
• Barium swallow shows narrowed distal end of esophagus; proximal dilatation and fluid appear high in esophagus; biopsy and cytology done to exclude cancer.

Continued

GI Disorders
Continued

ZENKER'S DIVERTICULUM (pulsion-type diverticulum)

Chief complaints
- *Pain:* scratchy throat
- *Nausea/vomiting:* regurgitation of food partially digested or eaten the day before
- *Dysphagia:* intermittent; progresses with continued eating

History
- Nocturnal coughing, halitosis, and weight loss are related signs and symptoms

Physical examination
- Protrusion on neck

Diagnostic studies
- Barium swallow shows pouching in upper esophagus; esophagoscopy performed to rule out other problems

---

ESOPHAGITIS

Chief complaints
- *Pain:* heartburn 1 hour after eating; aggravated by bending over, lying down, or straining; relieved by drinking or standing; pain may radiate to neck, arms, or jaws
- *Nausea/vomiting:* possible nocturnal regurgitation into mouth
- *Dysphagia:* Intermittent

History
- Hematemesis, melena, frequent eructation, increasing salivation, and nocturnal coughing are related signs and symptoms, aggravated by lying down.

Physical examination
- Physical signs usually absent.

Diagnostic studies
- Esophagoscopy shows eroded or ulcerated mucosa; cineroentgenography of esophagus with barium swallow shows weak peristalsis and failure of sphincter to relax.

ESOPHAGEAL CANCER

Chief complaints
- *Pain:* may be present under sternum, or in back or neck; progresses with advancing disease
- *Nausea/vomiting:* present in late stages
- *Dysphagia:* difficulty with solids, progressive difficulty with liquids

History
- Rapid weight loss and substernal burning after drinking hot fluids are related signs and symptoms.

Physical examination
- Cachexia, frequent coughing

Diagnostic studies
- Cytology shows cancer cells; barium swallow outlines tumor obstruction with irregular lesion; esophagoscopy visualizes lesion.

Continued

OTHER BODY SYSTEM DISORDERS

GI Disorders
Continued

PEPTIC ULCER

Chief complaint
• *Pain:* gnawing, burning pain more than 1 hour after eating; described as a feeling of nausea or hunger; relieved by eating; gastric ulcers may cause pain immediately after eating
History
• Emotional stress and drugs irritating to gastrointestinal (GI) tract; signs and symptoms occur in clusters, then subside and later recur.
Physical examination
• Abdominal tenderness
Diagnostic studies
• Upper GI series: crater easily visualized; endoscopy performed to confirm diagnosis; biopsy performed to rule out cancer; serum gastrin level elevated.

GASTRITIS (ACUTE AND CHRONIC)

Chief complaints
• *Pain:* epigastric pain slightly left of midline; indigestion
• *Nausea/vomiting:* if both present, hematemesis may occur
• *Constipation/diarrhea:* melena; diarrhea may occur
History
• Drug or chemical irritation, ingestion of irritating foods, alcoholism, pernicious anemia, severe stress, burns, surgery, trauma, and sepsis are predisposing factors.
Physical examination
• Abdominal tenderness
Diagnostic studies
• Fiberoptic endoscopy; mild leukocytosis; biopsy performed to diagnose chronic condition.

GASTROENTERITIS
(intestine also affected)

Chief complaints
• *Pain:* abdominal discomfort ranging from cramping to pain.
• *Nausea and vomiting:* both present
• *Constipation/diarrhea:* diarrhea
History
• Ingestion of infected food or water
• Travel to foreign country
• Ingestion of toxins: plants or toadstool
• Initiation of new drug therapy
Physical examination
• Fever; tender abdomen; borborygmi; signs of dehydration (thirst; poor skin turgor; flushed dry skin; coated tongue; irritability; confusion)
Diagnostic studies
• Stool culture or blood culture to identify causative bacteria or parasite.

Continued

GI Disorders
Continued

UPPER GASTROINTESTINAL (GI) BLEEDING (SECONDARY)

Chief complaints
• *Pain:* present; in ulcer disease, usually relieved by bleeding
• *Nausea/vomiting:* vomiting present; bright red from acute bleeding; dark red suggests past bleeding
• *Constipation/diarrhea:* bloody diarrhea with acute GI hemorrhage; melena with chronic upper GI bleeding

History
• Prior ulcer disease, alcoholism, and abuse of certain drugs.

Physical examination
• Weakness, fainting, orthostatic changes in blood pressure, tachycardia, diaphoresis

Diagnostic studies
• Hemoglobin and hematocrit measured to evaluate extent of blood loss; prothrombin time measured.

PERITONITIS

Chief complaints
• *Pain:* sudden, severe abdominal pain
• *Nausea/vomiting:* both present
• *Constipation/diarrhea:* inability to pass flatus or feces

History
• Abdominal distress, abdominal surgery, and traumatic abdominal injury are predisposing factors.

Physical examination
• Fever; abdominal ridigity; pallor; sweating; hypotension; thirst; tachycardia; shallow respirations; decreased bowel sounds; paralytic ileus causes resonance and tympany; rebound tenderness

Dianostic studies
• Leukocytosis; abdominal X-ray shows free gas and fluid in abdomen; paracentesis may reveal cause.

INTESTINAL OBSTRUCTION

Chief complaints
• *Pain:* colicky abdominal pain in epigastric or periumbilical area; in distal colon obstruction, pain referred to lumbar spine area
• *Nausea/vomiting:* in high obstruction, present; in large bowel obstruction, vomiting usually absent
• *Constipation/diarrhea:* in complete obstruction: constipation; in partial obstruction (for example, by tumor): pencil-thin stools; in obstruction caused by adhesions: diarrhea possible

History
• Family history of cancer is a predisposing factor; weight loss and weakness are related signs and symptoms.

Physical examination
• Abdominal distention and ten-
Continued

GI Disorders
Continued

INTESTINAL OBSTRUCTION
Continued

derness; paralytic ileus with absent bowel sounds; low-grade fever; possible palpable mass
Diagnostic studies
• Leukocytosis; X-ray shows distention; sigmoidoscopy and colonoscopy visualize obstruction; small intestine X-ray shows stepladder fluid and gas distribution.

DIVERTICULAR DISEASE (diverticulitis)

Chief complaints
• *Pain:* occasional lower left quadrant pain
• *Nausea/vomiting:* mild nausea present, but vomiting usually absent
• *Constipation/diarrhea:* constipation more common than diarrhea; occurs with onset of pain
History
• Long-term diet low in roughage and fiber is a predisposing factor.
Physical examination
• Low-grade fever; in severe disease, abdominal tenderness
Diagnostic studies
• Leukocytosis; flat plate abdominal view shows free air with perforation; barium enema visualizes diverticula.

ULCERATIVE COLITIS

Chief complaints
• *Pain:* cramping abdominal pain
• *Nausea/vomiting:* both present
• *Constipation/diarrhea:* profuse, episodic, bloody diarrhea with mucus possible
History
• Family history of disease and emotional stress are predisposing factors; weight loss and anorexia are related signs.
Physical examination
• Low-grade fever; abdominal tenderness
Diagnostic studies
• Leukocytosis; electrolyte imbalance; anemia; increased erythrocyte sedimentation rate; sigmoidoscopy shows increased friability and pus, mucus, and blood; barium enema shows extent of disease.

CROHN'S DISEASE

Chief complaints
• *Pain:* cramping lower right quadrant pain
• *Nausea/vomiting:* nausea present, but vomiting usually absent
• *Constipation/diarrhea:* mild, urgent diarrhea
History
• Family history of disease and emotional stress are predisposing
Continued

GI Disorders
Continued

CROHN'S DISEASE
Continued

factors; flatulence, weight loss, weakness, and malaise are related signs and symptoms.

Physical examination
• Low-grade fever; abdominal tenderness; possible mass in right lower quadrant

Diagnostic studies
• Leukocytosis; sigmoidoscopy usually negative; barium enema shows string sign (segments of stricture separated by normal bowel); biopsy confirms diagnosis.

COLORECTAL CANCER

Chief complaints
• *Pain:* abdominal cramping pain in later stages
• *Nausea/vomiting:* absent; present as the disease progresses
• *Constipation/diarrhea:* blood-streaked stools occur as early sign; pencil-thin stools possible; constipation alternating with diarrhea
• *Other:* weakness, fatigue, dyspnea, vertigo, anorexia, and weight loss

History
• Family history of cancer, polyposis, history of ulcerative colitis; malaise and loss of appetite.

Physical examination
• Weight loss; digital rectal examination may reveal palpable mass

Diagnostic studies
• Sigmoidoscopy, colonoscopy, and barium enema visualize tumor; biopsy reveals cancer cells.
• Intravenous pyelography verifies bilateral renal function and checks for any displacement of the kidneys, ureters, or bladder.
• Hemoccult test (guaiac) can detect blood in stools.

HEMORRHOIDS

Chief complaints
• *Pain:* occasional pain or bleeding on defecation; sudden, severe pain, if thrombosed
• *Nausea/vomiting:* absent
• *Constipation/diarrhea:* absent

History
• Prolonged sitting, vermiculation or pencil-thin stools, multiple pregnancies; changes in dietary intake; and straining when defecating.

Physical examination
• External hemorrhoids
• Grapelike clusters around anus; may be pink, red, or blue.

Diagnostic studies
• Proctoscopic or anoscopic examination reveals presence of tortuous, sac-like protrusions of the inferior, superior, or middle hemorrhoidal veins.
• Inspection reveals single or multiple grapelike vericosities.
• Digital examination of the rectum reveals internal hemorrhoids.

Other Related GI Disorders

APPENDICITIS

Chief complaints
• *Pain:* sudden epigastric or periumbilical pain; later localizes in right lower quadrant
• *Nausea/vomiting:* both present
• *Constipation/diarrhea:* diarrhea or, later, constipation
History
• Sudden onset of symptoms
Physical examination
• Mild fever, pain increases with right thigh extension, abdominal rigidity, rebound tenderness
Diagnostic studies
• White blood cell count elevated; X-ray may show local distention.

VIRAL HEPATITIS, TYPE A AND TYPE B

Chief complaints
• *Pain:* mild, constant pain in right upper quadrant
• *Nausea/vomiting:* nausea present; vomiting may be present
• *Constipation/diarrhea:* clay-colored stool may be present
History
• *Type A:* Contaminated food or water and contact with infected person are predisposing factors; *Type B:* transmitted parenterally or by infected secretions.
Physical examination
• Fever, chills, abdominal tenderness

Diagnostic studies
• SGOT and SGPT levels elevated; bilirubin level elevated; prolonged prothrombin time; serum albumin level low; serum globulin level elevated; antibody to hepatitis A virus confirms hepatitis A; hepatitis B surface antigens and hepatitis B antibodies confirm hepatitis B.

CIRRHOSIS

Chief complaints
• *Pain:* mild right upper quadrant pain; increasing as disease progresses
• *Nausea/vomiting:* both present
• *Constipation/diarrhea:* both present
History
• Alcoholism, hepatitis, heart failure, and hemochromatosis are predisposing factors; malaise, fatigue, anorexia leading to weight loss, pruritus, dark urine, and bleeding tendencies are related symptoms.
Physical examination
• Palpable liver and possibly spleen, jaundice, spider angiomas, peripheral edema; in progressive stages, ascites
Diagnostic studies
• Liver biopsy provides definitive diagnosis; serum glutamic-oxaloacetic transaminase (SGOT),

Continued

Other Related GI Disorders
Continued

CIRRHOSIS
Continued

serum glutamic-pyruvic transaminase (SGPT), and lactate dehydrogenase (LDH) levels elevated; serum alkaline phosphatase and bilrubin levels elevated, reflecting liver damage; prothrombin time and partial thromboplastin times may be prolonged.

CHOLECYSTITIS

Chief complaints
- *Pain:* onset sudden and severe
- *Nausea/vomiting:* both present
History
- Fatty food intolerance, indigestion, flatulence, and belching are related signs and symptoms; most common in obese, multiparous women over age 40
Physical examination
- Fever, abdominal tenderness in right upper quadrant, abdominal rigidity, palpable liver and gallbladder, tachycardia.
Diagnostic studies
- Cholecystography and ultrasound detect calculi; WBC may be elevated; serum alkaline phosphatase and bilirubin levels may be elevated.

PANCREATITIS (ACUTE AND CHRONIC)

Chief complaints
- *Pain:* constant epigastric pain; may radiate to back; pain worsened by lying down
- *Nausea/vomiting:* both present with bilious vomiting
- *Constipation/diarrhea:* absent
History
- Alcoholism, previous cholelithiasis, peptic ulcer, and use of drugs, such as azathioprine, are predisposing factors; pain aggravated by food or alcohol ingestion and restlessness are related symptoms.
Physical examination
- Mild fever, tachycardia, hypotension, abdominal distention, decreased bowel sounds, abdominal tenderness, and, if severe, abdominal rigidity and crackles at lung base
Diagnostic studies
- Serum amylase level elevated; marked leukocytosis; serum calcium level decreased; hyperglycemia; X-rays show distortion or edema of duodenal loop or calcification of pancreas.

Learning About Hepatitis

(HEPATITIS A VIRUS)

Contamination sources
- Raw shellfish
- Water
- Oral contact with fecal matter
- Blood and body secretions (in rare cases)

Incubation period
- 21 to 35 days; averages 30 days

Signs and symptoms (prodromal)
- Mental and physical fatigue
- Nausea; vomiting
- Anorexia
- Diarrhea
- Right upper quadrant pain from liver distention
- Headache
- Hives or skin rash
- Possible joint pain; arthritis in distal joints
- Angioneurotic edema (edema of skin, mucous membranes, and occasionally viscera)
- Elevated serum glutamic-oxaloacetic transaminase (SGOT) and serum glutamic-pyruvic transaminase (SGPT) levels 1 to 2 weeks prior to the appearance of jaundice
- Flulike symptoms, including sore throat, cough, irritated nasal mucous membrane, and fever of 100° to 104° F. (37.8° to 40° C.)

Signs and symptoms (icteric)
- Dark yellow urine, clay-colored stools, yellowish mucous membrane and sclerae (jaundice)
- Swollen lymph nodes, tender on palpation
- Weight loss (5 to 15 pounds)
- Moderately enlarged liver, tender on palpation
- Increased SGOT and SGPT levels
- Slightly increased alkaline phosphatase
- Prolonged prothrombin time
- Mild leukocytosis
- Bilirubinemia
- Bilirubin in urine, increased urobilinogen (above 4 mcg/24 hours)

Indications of recovery
- Gradual decrease of all symptoms. Stools, urine, skin, and sclerae return to normal color.
- Gradual return of normal lab values
- Recovery phase begins 1 to 2 weeks after jaundice subsides and usually lasts from 2 to 6 weeks.
- Return of appetite as patient begins to feel better

Continued

Learning About Hepatitis
Continued

(HEPATITIS B VIRUS)

Contamination sources
- Vaginal or anal intercourse
- Breast milk
- Syringes and needles
- Saliva
- Blood

Incubation period
- 60 to 150 days; averages 90 days

Signs and symptoms (prodromal)
- Low-grade fever of 100° to 101° F. (37.8° to 38.3° C.)
- Mental and physical fatigue
- Nausea; vomiting
- Anorexia
- Diarrhea
- Right upper quadrant pain from liver distention
- Headache
- Hives or skin rash
- Possible joint pain; arthritis in distal joints
- Angioneurotic edema (edema of skin, mucous membranes, and occasionally viscera)
- Elevated SGOT and SGPT levels 1 to 2 weeks prior to the appearance of jaundice
- Symptoms worse than Type A
- Diagnostic marker is presence of Hepatitis B Antigen (HBsAg), sometimes called Australian Antigen, in blood serum

Signs and symptoms (icteric)
- Same as Type A but more severe; possibly leading to massive liver necrosis and failure, and death

Indications of recovery
- Same as Type A

NON A NON B (VIRUS OTHER THAN A OR B)

Contamination sources
- Blood transfusions
- Syringes and needles

Incubation period
- 14 to 115 days

Signs and symptoms (prodromal)
- Mental and physical fatigue
- Nausea; vomiting
- Anorexia
- Diarrhea
- Right upper quadrant pain
- Headache
- Hives or skin rash
- Possible joint pain; arthritis in distal joints
- Angioneurotic edema
- Elevated SGOT and SGPT levels 1 to 2 weeks prior to the appearance of jaundice

Signs and symptoms (icteric)
- Same as Type A, except patient may not develop jaundice

Indications of recovery
- Same as Type A
- Recovery may last for months or may deteriorate to chronic hepatitis.

Learning About a Liver Biopsy

Wondering how a liver biopsy is performed? The doctor will insert a Vim-Silverman or modified Menghini needle into the right eighth or ninth intercostal space. Then, he'll extract a liver tissue sample and withdraw the needle. Such a biopsy is contraindicated if your patient has any of the following conditions: severe extrahepatic cholestasis; blood clotting problems; vascular malignant tumors; hepatic angiomas; congested liver, resulting from heart failure; or a hydatid cyst.

You're responsible for preparing your patient. Explain the procedure. Warn her that during the biopsy, and for a few days afterward, she'll feel some discomfort at the biopsy site.

Tell her she'll need to hold her breath for 5 to 10 seconds as the doctor inserts the needle. Holding her breath keeps her chest from moving and prevents a pleural cavity or diaphragm puncture.

Before the biopsy, obtain a sample of your patient's blood for type and cross match. Then, make sure a unit of the proper type blood's on hold, in case a transfusion is necessary. Also, withhold all food and oral fluids for 6 hours before the test.

Immediately before the procedure, tuck a pillow under your patient's right shoulder and back, and expose her right side. The doctor will prep the area with Betadine scrub. Then, he'll place a sterile fenestrated drape over the area.

After the procedure, apply a pressure bandage to the biopsy site. Tell your patient to lie on her right side for 2 hours after the test to splint the puncture site. Then, keep her on bed rest for the next 22 hours, or as ordered. Label and send the liver tissue specimen to the lab for analysis. Also, closely monitor your patient's vital signs.

In addition, check the injection site every 30 minutes for the first 4 hours after the biopsy, then hourly for the next 8 hours. If you see bleeding or a hematoma at the site, notify the doctor.

Document the procedure in your notes.

Paralytic (Adynamic) Ileus

Intestinal obstruction is the partial or complete blockage of the lumen in the small or large bowel. Small bowel obstruction is far more common (90% of patients) and usually more serious. Complete obstruction in any part of the bowel, if untreated, can cause death within hours from shock and vascular collapse. Intestinal obstruction is most likely to occur after abdominal surgery or in persons with congenital bowel deformities.

Paralytic ileus is a physiologic form of intestinal obstruction that usually develops in the small bowel after abdominal surgery. It causes decreased or absent intestinal motility that usually disappears spontaneously after 2 to 3 days. This condition can develop as a response to trauma, toxemia, or peritonitis, or as a result of electrolyte deficiencies (especially hypokalemia) and the use of certain drugs, such as ganglionic blocking agents and anticholinergics. It can also result from vascular causes, such as thrombosis or embolism. Excessive air swallowing may contribute to it, but paralytic ileus brought on by this factor alone seldom lasts more than 24 hours.

Clinical effects of paralytic ileus include severe abdominal distention, extreme distress, and possibly vomiting. The patient may be severely constipated or may pass flatus and small, liquid stools. Paralytic ileus lasting longer than 48 hours necessitates intubation for decompression and nasogastric suctioning. Because of the absence of peristaltic activity, a weighted Cantor tube may be necessary in the patient with extraordinary abdominal distention. However, such procedures must be used with extreme caution, because any additional trauma to the bowel can aggravate ileus. When paralytic ileus results from surgical manipulation of the bowel, treatment may also include cholinergic agents, such as neostigmine or bethanechol.

When caring for patients with paralytic ileus, warn those receiving cholinergic agents to expect certain paradoxical side effects, such as intestinal cramps and diarrhea. Remember that neostigmine produces cardiovascular side effects, usually bradycardia and hypotension. Check frequently for returning bowel sounds.

Recognizing Hepatic Coma

Patients in hepatic coma (hepatic encephalopathy) progress through the following four stages, with accompanying clinical features:

- *Prodromal:* mild confusion, euphoria or depression, vacant stare, inappropriate laughter, forgetfulness, inability to concentrate, slow mentation, slurred speech, untidiness, lethargy, belligerence, minimal asterixis (flapping tremor).

  Watch carefully for these subtle symptoms. These are not necessarily present at the same time.

- *Impending:* obvious obtundation, aberrant behavior, definite asterixis, constructional apraxia.

  To test for asterixis (flapping tremor), have the patient raise both arms, with forearms flexed and fingers extended. To test for constructional apraxia, keep a serial record of the patient's handwriting and figure construction, and check it for progressive deterioration.

- *Stuporous* (patient can still be aroused): marked confusion, incoherent speech, asterixis, noisiness, abusiveness, violence, definitely abnormal EEG.

  Restraints may be necessary at this stage. *Do not sedate the patient; sedation could be fatal.*

- *Comatose* (patient cannot be aroused, responds only to painful stimuli): no asterixis but positive Babinski's sign, hepatic fetor (breath has musty, sweet odor), and elevated serum ammonia level.

  Degree of hepatic fetor correlates with the degree of somnolence and confusion.

Diagnosing Hepatic Coma

Clinical features, a positive history of liver disease, and elevated serum ammonia levels in venous and arterial samples confirm hepatic encephalopathy. Other supportive lab values include EEG, elevated bilirubin, and prolonged prothrombin time.

OTHER BODY SYSTEM DISORDERS

Common Inflammatory and/or Infectious Disorders

ORCHITIS

Chief complaints
- *Changes in voiding patterns:* usually none
- *Penile discharge:* usually none
- *Scrotal or inguinal mass:* unilateral or bilateral scrotal swelling
- *Pain or tenderness:* varies from slight discomfort to extreme pain in one or both testes
- *Impotence:* precipitated by pain
- *Infertility:* possible with severe bilateral infection as with mumps

History
- Prior infection, especially epididymitis or mumps

Physical examination and diagnostic studies
- Fever, possibly nausea and vomiting
- Inspection reveals reddened scrotal skin, swollen testes
- Palpation reveals warm scrotal skin, tender testes
- Complete blood count reveals elevated WBC count

PROSTATITIS

Chief complaints
- *Changes in voiding patterns:* frequency, urgency; nocturia and hesitancy possible
- *Penile discharge:* if condition is acute, thin, watery, blood-streaked semen possible
- *Scrotal or inguinal mass:* none
- *Pain or tenderness:* dysuria common; possibly lower back pain and/or perineal pressure; painful ejaculation possible
- *Impotence:* decreased libido and potency possible
- *Infertility:* possible

History
- Chronic form commonly occurs in young men
- Prior ascending urinary tract infection common

Physical examination and diagnostic studies
- Rectal palpation reveals, in acute form, firm, enlarged, tender, boggy prostate gland; in chronic form, enlarged prostate possible, as well as firmness due to prostatic calculi
- Fever and chills possible in acute form
- Third specimen of three- or four-glass urine test contains many WBCs

Continued

Common Inflammatory and/or Infectious Disorders
Continued

EPIDIDYMITIS

Chief complaints
• *Changes in voiding patterns:* usually none; frequency occurs if urinary tract infection is present
• *Penile discharge:* usually none
• *Scrotal or inguinal mass:* unilateral or bilateral scrotal swelling
• *Pain or tenderness:* intense scrotal pain; may radiate to rectum, lower back, suprapubic region
• *Impotence:* precipitated by pain
• *Infertility:* possible with severe bilateral infection
History
• Prior urinary tract infection may be present
Physical examination and diagnostic studies
• Fever, chills, malaise, and weakness
• Inspection reveals enlarged epididymis, reddened, tender, and swollen scrotal skin
• Palpation reveals warm scrotal skin, painful epididymis
• Hardened scrotal contents
• May be accompanied by cystitis
• Complete blood count reveals elevated WBC count
• Urinalysis may show pyuria
• Gait may resemble duck waddle to limit scrotal discomfort

GONORRHEA

Chief complaints
• *Changes in voiding patterns:* usually none, but frequency and urgency of urination possible
• *Penile discharge:* present; thick, yellow, and a creamy consistency, but may start as a serous milky white secretion
• *Scrotal or inguinal mass:* tender; lymphadenopathy possible
• *Pain or tenderness:* dysuria
• *Impotence:* may be temporary, secondary to dysuria
• *Infertility:* present only if untreated (in advanced stage secondary to scar tissue formation in epididymis)
History
• Sexual exposure within preceding 2 weeks
• Incubation period 2 to 5 days but symptoms may not appear for 3 months
Physical examination and diagnostic studies
• Edematous urethral meatus possible
• Enlarged, tender or reddened penis
• Gram-negative intracellular diplococci on stained smear of urethral exudate
• Positive culture on Thayer-Martin medium or equivalent

Continued

Common Inflammatory and/or Infectious Disorders
Continued

SYPHILITIC CHANCRE

Chief complaints
- *Changes in voiding patterns:* none in early stage
- *Penile discharge:* none
- *Scrotal or inguinal mass:* enlarged inguinal lymph nodes possible
- *Pain or tenderness:* none
- *Impotence:* none
- *Infertility:* usually none if detected and treated early

History
- Caused by sexual relations with infected partner

Physical examination and diagnostic studies
- Oval or round indurated ulcer with raised edge
- Dark-field microscopic examination of exudate confirms diagnosis
- Lesion usually found on the penis, may occur on the anus-rectal area or on the oropharynx.
- Lesion may disappear in 10 to 40 days if untreated and progresses to the next stage.

GENITAL HERPES

Chief complaints
- *Changes in voiding patterns:* none
- *Penile discharge:* none
- *Scrotal or inguinal mass:* tender, enlarged inguinal lymph nodes
- *Pain or tenderness:* painful lesions during ulcerative stage; dysuria possible
- *Impotence:* none
- *Infertility:* usually none

History
- Caused by sexual relations with infected partner

Physical examination and diagnostic studies
- Single or multiple, fluid-filled lesion usually on the glans penis, penile shaft, or foreskin
- Extragenital lesions may appear on the mouth or anus (may lead to rare complications such as herpetic keratitis, causing blindness, and potentially fatal herpetic encephalitis)
- Urethral discharge
- Shallow ulcerative lesions, with local redness and swelling when ruptured
- Fever and malaise
- Localized pain and burning
- Tissue culture may reveal herpes simplex Type 2 in vesical fluid

Noninflammatory Benign Conditions

BENIGN PROSTATIC HYPERTROPHY

Chief complaints
- *Changes in voiding patterns:* urinary hesitancy, intermittency with dribbling; reduced urinary stream caliber and force; straining; possibly retention
- *Penile discharge:* none
- *Scrotal or inguinal mass:* none
- *Pain or tenderness:* burning on urination with cystitis if accompanied by urinary tract infection
- *Impotence:* possible if nerves innervating penis are damaged during open prostatectomy
- *Infertility:* common following transurethral prostatectomy due to retrograde ejaculation

History
- Commonly occurs in men over age 50

Physical examination and diagnostic studies
- Nocturia
- Inability to void after exposure to cold or consumption of alcohol.
- Rectal palpation reveals a firm, slightly elastic, enlarged, smooth prostate, with varying degrees of tenderness; rectal mucosa easily glides over hypertrophied gland
- Cystourethroscopy shows prostatic encroachment on the urethra and effects of enlargement on bladder
- Cytology examination reveals whether changes are benign or malignant.
- Urinalysis shows presence of red cells and infection

VARICOCELE

Chief complaints
- *Changes in voiding patterns:* none
- *Penile discharge:* none
- *Scrotal or inguinal mass:* present in scrotum, usually on left side
- *Pain or tenderness:* no acute pain or tenderness; some discomfort caused by size of mass
- *Impotence:* none
- *Infertility:* none

History
- Common in males of high school or college age

Physical examination and diagnostic studies
- Inspection reveals lower-hanging testis on affected side, pendulous and irregular scrotum
- Palpation reveals soft, irregular mass; enlarged veins make the patient's scrotum feel like a bag of worms

Continued

Noninflammatory Benign Conditions
Continued

HYDROCELE

Chief complaints
- *Changes in voiding patterns:* usually none
- *Penile discharge:* none
- *Scrotal or inguinal mass:* present in scrotum
- *Pain or tenderness:* usually none, except with very large mass
- *Impotence:* none
- *Infertility:* none

History
- Common in infants and adults
- Prior infection of testis, epididymitis possible
- May occur from localized trauma or systemic infectious diseases, such as mumps, pharyngitis and tuberculosis

Physical examination and diagnostic studies
- Inspection reveals smooth, fluctuant mass in scrotum of pyriform or globular shape, with large end above; frequently has consistency of a testicle and may give the appearance of three testicles contained within the scrotum; transilluminates as a translucent mass
- Palpation reveals mass that cannot be reduced into abdomen; doesn't transmit cough impulse.
- May accompany testicular tumors

SCROTAL HERNIA

Chief complaints
- *Changes in voiding patterns:* none
- *Penile discharge:* none
- *Scrotal or inguinal mass:* present in scrotum (extension of inguinal hernia)
- *Pain or tenderness:* usually none although mild, aching discomfort possible
- *Impotence:* none
- *Infertility:* none

History
- Heavy lifting that increases intraabdominal pressure

Physical examination and diagnostic studies
- Inspection reveals inguinoscrotal mass that doesn't transilluminate.
- Palpation reveals inguinoscrotal mass that transmits cough impulse; possible to reduce mass into abdomen
- Auscultation may detect bowel sounds in the scrotum

Cancers

CANCER OF THE TESTIS

Chief complaints
- *Changes in voiding patterns:* none in early stage
- *Penile discharge:* none
- *Scrotal or inguinal mass:* testicular mass present
- *Pain or tenderness:* usually none until late stages, when accompanied by a feeling of heaviness or an aching or dragging sensation in groin
- *Impotence:* psychogenic impotence possible
- *Infertility:* none

History
- Common in men between ages 20 and 40

Physical examination and diagnostic studies
- Gynecomastia
- Inspection and palpation reveal firm, nontender testicular mass; doesn't transilluminate
- Biopsy confirms diagnosis
- Serum alpha-fetoprotein and beta human chorionic gonadotropin provide important information about tumor type and activity
- Enlargement, swelling, or hardening of the testis
- In young males, precocious genital and body development

CANCER OF THE PROSTATE

Chief complaints
- *Changes in voiding patterns:* in later stages, urinary hesitancy, dribbling, and possibly retention
- *Penile discharge:* usually none
- *Scrotal or inguinal mass:* none
- *Pain or tenderness:* lower back, hip, and leg pain common in advanced state, caused by metastases to the bones of the pelvis and spine
- *Impotence:* follows radical resection of prostate
- *Infertility:* follows radical resection of prostate

History
- More common in black men over age 50
- Incidence increases with advancing age

Physical examination and diagnostic studies
Rectal palpation reveals hard, irregular nodule on posterior prostate; becomes fixed as lesion progresses
- Biopsy confirms diagnosis; serum acid phosphatase level elevated when tumor spreads beyond prostatic capsule
- Cytology study reveals whether changes are benign or malignant
- Tumors metastasize to bones, brain, and lung

Common Inflammatory and/or Infectious Disorders

MONILIA (CANDIDIASIS)

Chief complaints
• *Discharge:* heavy, with yeasty, sweet odor for preceding 3 to 4 days
• *Pain:* dysuria
• *Pruritus:* present, with itching
History
• Predisposing factors include increased emotional stress, birth control pill use, pregnancy, diabetes mellitus, antibiotic or steroid therapy, severe illness
• Premenstrual onset
• Episodes recur, may lead to chronic cervicitis and erosion
• If untreated, may lead to excoriation and secondary infection
Physical examination and diagnostic studies
• White, curdlike, profuse discharge on vulva, vagina, and cervix; erythema; pruritus; edema of vulvovaginal area
• Culture; wet smear with 10% potassium hydroxide to confirm diagnosis

HEMOPHILUS VAGINALIS

Chief complaints
• *Discharge:* fishy odor; gray to yellow-white; soaks through clothing; may last for months
• *Pain:* little or none

History
• Predisposing factors include frequent sexual activity, birth control pill use, frequent douching, sex with partner who doesn't use condom
• Episodes recur, leading to cervical erosion
• If untreated, may lead to contact dermatitis and secondary infection
Physical examination and diagnostic studies
• Wet smear (clue cells) identifies organism

PUBIC LICE

Chief complaint
• *Pruritus:* severe itching of genital hair areas for several days
History
• Predisposing factors include frequent sexual activity and household history of lice.
• Lice transferred primarily by direct contact.
• Infection of any hairy part of body possible.
Physical examination and diagnostic studies
• Oval, light-colored swellings near base of hair shafts; freckled, erythematous, scratched, petechial and/or edematous skin under pubic hair; lice ova (nits) make pubic hair feel bumpy and irregular

Continued

OTHER BODY SYSTEM DISORDERS

Common Inflammatory and/or Infectious Disorders
Continued

TRICHOMONIASIS

Chief complaints
• *Discharge:* frothy, green-yellow, malodorous, profuse
• *Pain:* possible vaginal soreness, burning, dyspareunia
• *Pruritus:* vaginal itching
History
• Predisposing factors include prior pregnancy, sex with partner who doesn't use condom, close contact with infected person
• Premenstrual onset
• Most common in females of childbearing age
• Complications may include urinary tract infection, inflammation of Skene's and Bartholin's glands, increased cervical cancer risk
Physical examination and diagnostic studies
• Erythema and edema of vulva and vagina
• Raised petechial lesions on vagina and cervix
• Wet-mount smear of vaginal secretions made with physiologic saline (motile protozoa)

GONORRHEA

Chief complaints
• *Discharge:* slight to profuse, purulent (vaginal and urethral)
• *Pain:* dysuria; pelvic or abdominal discomfort
• *Pruritus:* may be present
History
• Frequent sexual activity is a predisposing factor
• Frequently asymptomatic until ascending infection occurs
• Most common in females in their teens and twenties
• Complications include urethritis, bartholinitis, proctitis, salpingitis, pharyngitis, stomatitis, and conjunctivitis
• If untreated, may lead to systemic infection, including pelvic inflammatory disease, skin eruptions on trunk and legs, arthritis, and tendonitis
Physical examination and diagnostic studies
• Fever; skin lesions; arthritis
• Urethral meatus may be erythematous and, when milked, may exude pus
• Cervix may be reddened and edematous
• Gram's stain smear for gram-negative diplococci; culture on Thayer-Martin media to confirm diagnosis

ATROPHIC VAGINITIS

Chief complaints
• *Discharge:* follows intercourse or long walks

Continued

Common Inflammatory and/or Infectious Disorders
Continued

ATROPHIC VAGINITIS
Continued

• *Pain:* vaginal burning and soreness; postcoital discomfort and dyspareunia possible
• *Abnormal uterine bleeding:* spotting possible after douching or after intercourse
• *Pruritus:* vaginal itching
History
• Predisposing factors include bilateral oophorectomy and cessation of estrogen therapy
• Postmenopausal onset
• If untreated, may lead to secondary infection, altered sexual self-esteem, and possibly marital discord and depressive reaction
Physical examination and diagnostic studies
• Dry vulva, possibly vulvitis, friable mucosa, few or absent vaginal rugae, pale and shiny vaginal mucosa, and small and tender cervix

PRIMARY SYPHILIS

Chief complaints
• *Discharge:* none
• *Pain:* none
• *Lumps, masses, ulcerations:* solitary, hard, oval ulcer (chancre) on vulva, perineum, labia, cervix, and possibly breasts, fingers, lips, oral mucosa, tongue for several days to weeks
• *Pruritus:* none
History
• Frequent sexual activity
• May be asymptomatic between stages
Physical examination and diagnostic studies
• Enlarged inguinal lymph nodes possible
• Fluorescent treponemal antibody absorption test and darkfield examination for syphilis

FOREIGN-BODY VAGINITIS

Chief complaints
• *Discharge:* purulent and fetid, lasting about 1 week
• *Pain:* vaginal
History
• Predisposing factors include pessary, tampon, or diaphragm use; emotional instability; memory instability; inadequate sex education; use of intravaginal object for sexual pleasure.
• Complications include vaginal fistula, cervical erosion, and adhesions
Physical examination and diagnostic studies
• Obstructing mass in vagina
• Possible laceration of cervix or vaginal mucosa
• Culture taken

Continued

Common Inflammatory and/or Infectious Disorders
Continued

GENITAL HERPES II

Chief complaints
• *Discharge:* watery; accompanies appearance of lesions
• *Pain:* blisters and/or sores for preceding 1 or 2 days; prodromal symptoms of burning or tingling in genital area possible; *may* be asymptomatic; severe vulval pain following appearance of lesions; severe dysuria or retention possible
• *Lumps, masses, ulcerations:* blisters and ulcers covering extensive areas of the vulva and the perianal skin
• *Pruritus:* mild itching in genital area preceding eruption of lesions

History
• Most common in women from late teens to early thirties
• Predisposing factors include recent gynecologic or lower urinary tract examination, frequent sexual activity, sex with partner who doesn't use condom, recurrent infection
• If untreated, primary lesions persist for 3 to 6 weeks and heal spontaneously
• Symptoms of fever, malaise, or anorexia possible 3 to 7 days after exposure
• Complications include fever; enlarged, tender inguinal lymph nodes; urinary retention, leading to urinary tract infection; cervical cancer; spontaneous abortion or premature delivery; severely infected newborn if delivered vaginally; possibly viremia

Physical examination and diagnostic studies
• Cervix may be covered with yellow-gray film; urethra, bladder, and vulva may be extremely tender
• Culture of vesicle or ulcer fluid; Tzanck test confirms diagnosis

BARTHOLINITIS (BARTHOLIN ADENITIS)

Chief complaints
• *Pain:* present in Bartholin's gland; reddened, tender overlying skin
• *Lumps, masses, ulcerations:* large lump on one side of genitalia for several days

History
• Predisposing factors include frequent sexual activity and use of feminine hygiene product
• Abscess or chronic infection possible

Physical examination and diagnostic studies
• Tender, hot, posterior labium with hard swelling and no purulent drainage
• Culture taken

Continued

Common Inflammatory and/or Infectious Disorders
Continued

CHLAMYDIA

Chief complaints
- *Discharge:* purulent, rare
- *Pain:* dysuria

History
- Predisposing factors include frequent sexual activity and sex with partner who doesn't use condom
- Most common in women in their teens or twenties
- Usually asymptomatic
- Complications include trachoma, conjunctivitis, lymphogranuloma venereum, cervical cancer (long-term), salpingitis, newborn conjunctivitis and pneumonia, postpartum endometritis.

Physical examination and diagnostic studies
- Rough cervical patches; thickened cervix possible but not common
- Culture taken; antibody titer urinalysis performed

CONDYLOMATA ACUMINATA (VENEREAL WARTS)

Chief complaints
- *Pain:* usually painless but pruritic unless warts become infected or irritated by friction; intercourse may be painful if condylomata are large and/or extensive
- *Lumps, masses, ulcerations:* soft warts on perineal and perianal areas

History
- May accompany trichomoniasis; resembles vulval cancer
- Predisposing factors include frequent sexual activity, birth control pill use, pregnancy, massive immunosuppressive therapy, sex with partner who doesn't use condom

Physical examination and diagnostic studies
- Inspection reveals soft, wartlike, irregularly shaped growths on vulva and perineum and in perianal, vaginal, and/or cervical areas; in advanced stage, cauliflower or deep rose-colored lesions
- Dark-field examination of scrapings from wart cells shows marked vascularization of epidermal cells

ACUTE PELVIC INFLAMMATORY DISEASE (PID)

Chief complaints
- *Discharge:* history of vaginal discharge of variable duration
- *Pain:* sharp, bilateral, and cramping, usually in lower quadrants
- *Abnormal uterine bleeding:* irregular and/or longer, heavier menstrual periods   *Continued*

Common Inflammatory and/or Infectious Disorders
Continued

PID *Continued*

History
- With PID: history of recent abortion, intrauterine device use, sexually transmitted disease, dysuria, severe dysmenorrhea; with acute PID: nausea, vomiting, and elevated temperature
- If untreated, acute PID becomes chronic, causing peritoneal abscess, massive adhesions, and sterility
- PID may be confused with ruptured appendix, ectopic pregnancy, or perforation of gastrointestinal abscesses

Physical examination and diagnostic studies
- Pelvic examination reveals tender cervix; bilateral adnexal enlargement, tenderness, immobility
- Culture of *Streptococcus* or *Neisseria gonorrhoeae*

TOXIC SHOCK SYNDROME (TSS)

Chief complaint
- *Pain:* abdominal; myalgia, arthralgia, headache

History
- History of tampon use during active vaginal bleeding; early recognition depends on knowledge of patient's history of tampon use and hygiene, last menstrual period, past menstrual history, and previous episodes of TSS
- More common in females
- May be confused with any viral systemic illness

Physical examination and diagnostic studies
- Temperature over 102° F. (38.9° C.), nausea, vomiting, hypotension, photophobia, abdominal pain, myalgia, arthralgia, headache
- Culture of *Staphylococcus aureus* from vagina

MASTITIS

Chief complaints
- *Pain:* present, accompanied by tenderness in breast
- *Lumps, masses, ulcerations:* hard, reddened breast

History
- Usually occurs third or fourth week postpartum; nipples usually cracked
- If untreated, may evolve into breast abscess with palpable fluctuance and painful axillary lymphadenopathy

Physical examination and diagnostic studies
- Firm, tender, warm and reddened area apparent in affected breast
- Culture usually yields offending organism: *Staphylococcus aureus*

Common Noninflammatory Benign Lesions

CYSTOCELE (SEVERAL DE-
GREES)

Chief complaints
• *Pain:* dysuria, with infection,
back pain
• *Lumps, masses, ulcerations:*
fullness at vaginal opening
History
• Predisposing factors include
multiparity, obesity, chronic ascites, prolonged labors, instru-
ment deliveries, chronic cough,
heavy-object lifting
• Symptoms may result in social
withdrawal, depression
• May be asymptomatic
Physical examination and diag-
nostic studies
• Inspection reveals soft, reduci-
ble, mucosal mass bulging into
anterior introitus; with Valsalva's
maneuver, the mass increases
and urine may squirt or dribble
from meatus
• Laboratory tests include urinalysis

RECTOCELE (SEVERAL DE-
GREES)

Chief complaints
• *Pain:* backaches possible
• *Lumps, masses, ulcerations:*
fullness at vaginal opening

History
• Predisposing factors include
multiparity, obesity, chronic ascites, prolonged labors, instru-
ment deliveries, chronic cough,
heavy-object lifting
• May be accompanied by
chronic constipation, laxative and
enema dependency, iatrogenic
diarrhea
• Most common in postmenopausal women
Physical examination and diag-
nostic studies
• Inspection reveals mass bulging
into posterior introitus.

PROLAPSED UTERUS (SEV-
ERAL DEGREES)

Chief complaints
• *Pain:* heaviness in pelvis
• *Lumps, masses, ulcerations:*
feels as if she's sitting on a ball
• *Abnormal uterine bleeding:*
menometrorrhagia
History
• Predisposing factors include
those for cystocele and rectocele,
as well as history of sacral nerve
disorders, diabetic neuropathy,
and pelvic tumors
• Commonly associated with cystocele and rectocele
• Commonly accompanied by urinary tract infection, constipation,
and painful defecation but may be
asymptomatic   *Continued*

Common Noninflammatory Benign Lesions
Continued

Physical examination and diagnostic studies
- Cervix palpable, closer to introitus, and can be pushed in caudally; in advanced stage, mucosa of exposed mass outside introitus is ulcerated and friable.

ENDOMETRIOSIS

Chief complaints
- *Pain:* menstrual; referred to the rectum and lower sacral or coccygeal regions; dyspareunia probable with uterosacral involvement or vaginal extension; pain on defecation with uterosacral involvement or vaginal extension; dysuria possible
- *Abnormal uterine bleeding:* excessive, prolonged, or frequent, with no specific pattern

History
- Most common in women ages 25 to 45
- History of menstrual disturbances
- Commonly accompanied by constipation, pain with defecation during menstruation, infertility

Physical examination and diagnostic studies
- Multiple tender nodules palpable along the uterosacral ligaments or in the rectovaginal septum of the posterior fornix of the vagina
- Diagnosis can be confirmed

only by visualization of the lesion; accomplished directly with external lesions, or by laparotomy or endoscopy with internal lesions
- Uterus may be fixed in retroposition; attempts to move it accompanied by severe pain
- Endometrial cysts present as irregular enlargement of ovary

UTERINE LEIOMYOMAS (FIBROIDS AND MYOMAS)

Chief complaints
- *Pain:* in pelvic area; accompanied by dysmenorrhea or sensation of weight
- *Lumps, masses, ulcerations:* lump in lower abdomen possible; with large tumors, general enlargement of abdomen
- *Abnormal uterine bleeding:* excessive menstrual flow and/or irregular bleeding

History
- History of involuntary infertility or repeat spontaneous abortion
- Accompanying symptoms include irritability, increased frequency of urination, possibly dysuria, constipation, and occasionally pain on defecation

Physical examination and diagnostic studies
- Bimanual examination may reveal one or more nodular outgrowths on the uterine surface or within the uterine wall

Continued

Common Noninflammatory Benign Lesions
Continued

FUNCTIONAL OVARIAN CYSTS (FOLLICLE CYSTS, CORPUS LUTEUM CYSTS)

Chief complaints
• *Pain:* with large follicle cysts, mild pelvic discomfort, lower back pain, or deep dyspareunia possible; with corpus luteum cysts, localized pain and tenderness
• *Abnormal uterine bleeding:* with follicle cysts, occasional menstrual irregularities; with corpus luteum cysts, late menstrual periods, followed by persistent bleeding
History
• Most common in women ages 20 to 40
• May be asymptomatic
Physical examination and diagnostic studies
• Bimanual palpation may reveal presence of cyst
• Laparoscopy or laparotomy may be performed to confirm diagnosis

FIBROCYSTIC DISEASE OF THE BREAST (MAMMARY DYSPLASIA, CYSTIC ADENOSIS, CHRONIC CYSTIC DISEASE, CYSTIC MASTITIS)

Chief complaints
• *Discharge:* may be slight
• *Pain:* cyst pain and tenderness possible, especially in premenstrual phase of cycle
• *Lumps, masses, ulcerations:* thickened, nodular areas in breast
History
• Most common in women during reproductive years
• May be exacerbated by caffeine intake
Physical examination and diagnostic studies
• Palpation of breast reveals single or multiple masses; usually bilateral, mobile, well-defined, and tender
• Diagnosis established by aspiration of cysts or by biopsy

MAMMARY DUCT ECTASIA

Chief complaints
• *Discharge:* from nipple, accompanied by nipple retraction
• *Pain:* in affected areas
• *Lumps, masses, ulcerations:* rubbery lesions in breasts; inflammation
History
• Most common in early-stage–menopausal and menopausal women
Physical examination and diagnostic studies
• Inspection reveals nipple discharge and, possibly, nipple retraction
• Palpation reveals subareolar ducts as rubbery lesions filled with a pastelike material; enlarged regional lymph nodes possible

Common Malignant Diseases

ENDOMETRIAL CANCER

Chief complaints
- *Pain:* present in later, invasive stages of disease
- *Abnormal uterine bleeding:* spotting for days to months; may go undetected

History
- History of previous estrogen therapy, nulliparousness, obesity, and possibly diabetes, hypertension, or previous curettage, sterility, or fertility problems
- Most common in menopausal or postmenopausal women

Physical examination and diagnostic studies
- Inspection usually reveals brown or red stain on crotch of clothing; possibly cervical lesion
- Palpation may reveal uterus or adnexal mass, usually nontender
- Laboratory tests include tissue examination by dilatation and curettage or by section biopsy

OVARIAN CARCINOMA

Chief complaints
- *Pain:* abdominal, in later stage of disease
- *Lumps, masses, ulcerations:* mass in lower abdomen; may be first indication of disease; ascites possible
- *Abnormal uterine bleeding:* irregular or postmenopausal bleeding possible but infrequent

History
- History of urinary frequency and constipation possible
- Most common in early-stage–menopausal or postmenopausal, nulliparous women
- Usually asymptomatic in early stages
- May be secondary site of cancer

Physical examination and diagnostic studies
- Lower genital tract usually normal, but displaced cervix possible
- Bimanual palpation usually delineates ovarian mass; malignant tumors are bilateral and partly solid

Continued

Common Malignant Diseases
Continued

CARCINOMA OF CERVIX IN SITU (PREINVASIVE)

Chief complaints
• *Pain:* absent
• *Lumps, masses, ulcerations:* absent
• *Abnormal uterine bleeding:* absent

History
• Predisposing factors include sexual activity before age 20, continued exposure to multiple sexual partners, frequent vaginal infections, genital herpes
• Usually asymptomatic

Physical examination and diagnostic studies
• Lesion frequently overlooked; friable cervix and erosions or superficial defect of the ectocervix possible
• Laboratory tests include Pap test, colposcopy, microscopic examination of biopsy specimen

BREAST CANCER

Chief complaints
• *Discharge:* from nipple, usually bloody
• *Pain:* absent; breast pain possible but not common
• *Lumps, masses, ulcerations:* lump in breast

History
• Most common in white women of middle or upper socioeconomic class and over age 35, and in those with a family history of breast cancer
• History of long menstrual cycles; early menses or late menopause; first pregnancy after age 35; endometrial or ovarian cancer

Physical examination and diagnostic studies
• Inspection may reveal enlarged, shrunken, or dimpled breast, with nipple erosion, retraction, and/or discharge; abnormality may not be obvious
• Palpation reveals lump, which is usually nontender, firm or hard, irregularly shaped and fixed to skin or fixed to underlying tissues; enlarged surrounding lymph nodes possible
• Laboratory tests include mammography, biopsy, and thermography

Determining Uterine Positions

You can accurately determine uterine position while performing a bimanual examination. Use this chart as a guide to evaluate your findings.

ANTEVERTED

Cervix position
Anterior vaginal wall
Palpability of body and fundus
Palpable with one hand on the patient's abdomen and the fingers of the other hand in her vagina

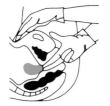

RETROVERTED

Cervix position
Posterior vaginal wall
Palpability of body and fundus
Not palpable

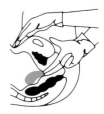

MIDPOSITION

Cervix position
Vaginal apex
Palpability of body and fundus
May not be palpable

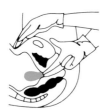

ANTEFLEXED

Cervix position
Anterior vaginal wall or apex
Palpability of body and fundus
Easily palpable (angulation of the isthmus felt in anterior fornix)

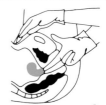

Continued

Determining Uterine Positions
Continued

RETROFLEXED

Cervix position
Anterior or posterior vaginal wall
or apex
Palpability of body and fundus
Not palpable

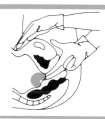

Performing a Bimanual Vaginal Examination

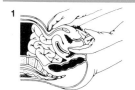

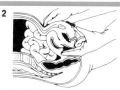

1 To palpate the uterus and anterior fornix, direct your index and middle fingers toward the patient's anterior fornix. In this position you should feel part of the anterior uterine wall. Place your other hand on the abdomen, just above the symphysis pubis, to palpate the posterior uterine wall.

2 To palpate the posterior fornix, direct your index and middle fingers toward the patient's posterior fornix. Press upward and forward so that you can palpate the ante-

rior uterine wall with your abdominally placed hand.

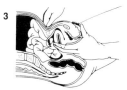

3 To palpate the adnexa, direct your index and middle fingers toward the patient's right lateral fornix and place your other hand on the patient's lower right quadrant. Palpate right and left sides.

Pregnancy Disorders

HISTORY AND CHIEF COMPLAINTS	PHYSICAL EXAMINATION AND DIAGNOSTIC STUDIES
Gestational edema • Signs and symptoms include generalized fluid accumulation after 12 hours of bed rest	• Edema (+ 1 pitting) • After bed rest, weight gain of 5 lb (2.26 kg) or more in 1 week with or without edema
Chronic hypertensive disease • History of hypertension before pregnancy, and/or hypertension apparent before 20th week of gestation • No history of neoplastic trophoblastic disease or persistent hypertension after 6 weeks postpartum in previous pregnancies	• Systolic blood pressure: 140 mm Hg or greater, or rise of 30 mm Hg or greater from baseline pressure • Diastolic blood pressure: 90 mm Hg or greater, or rise of 15 mm Hg or greater from baseline pressure
Gestational hypertension • No past history of hypertension	• May not occur until the first 24 hours postpartum and disappears within 10 days postpartum • Blood pressure as described in chronic hypertensive disease; usually discovered on physical examination during latter half of pregnancy • No other signs of preeclampsia or hypertensive vascular disease
Gestational proteinuria • No history of hypertension, edema, renal infection, or known renovascular disease	• Urine protein level increased by 0.3 g/liter in 24-hour period, or 1 g/liter in two different specimens collected at least 6 hours apart

Continued

Pregnancy Disorders
Continued

HISTORY AND CHIEF COMPLAINTS	PHYSICAL EXAMINATION AND DIAGNOSTIC STUDIES

Preeclampsia
- Occurs after 20th week of gestation; may appear earlier with an advanced hydatidiform mole or with extensive molar change; most common in primigravidas, especially older women and pregnant adolescents
- Family history of preeclampsia or eclampsia
- Signs and symptoms include visual disturbances ranging from blurred vision to blindness in extreme cases, and headache (usually mild; uncommon)
- May be asymptomatic except for elevated blood pressure
- With severe preeclampsia, signs and symptoms include nausea, vomiting, irritability, severe frontal headache, epigastric or right upper quadrant pain (usually a sign of impending seizure), and respiratory distress suggesting pulmonary edema

- Edema evidenced by puffiness of fingers and swollen eyelids; becomes generalized and is also apparent in sacral area and abdominal wall; sudden, excessive weight gain; hypertension; proteinuria
- With severe preeclampsia, increased blood pressure (160/110 mm Hg) that does not decrease with bed rest; proteinuria (urine protein increased 5 g in 24 hours, +3 or +4), oliguria (urinary output reduced by 500 ml or more in 24 hours); increased serum creatine, cerebral disturbances, hyperreflexia (3 to 4 +/4 +, clonus), cyanosis, severe thrombocytopenia, hepatocellular damage

Superimposed preeclampsia or eclampsia
- Predisposing factors include chronic hypertensive vascular disease or renal disease
- May occur early in pregnancy and progress to eclampsia

- Same as preeclampsia and eclampsia

Continued

Pregnancy Disorders
Continued

HISTORY AND CHIEF COMPLAINTS	PHYSICAL EXAMINATION AND DIAGNOSTIC STUDIES
Eclampsia • Most common in last trimester • Family history of preeclampsia or eclampsia • Signs and symptoms usually preceded by preeclampsia; in the absence of neurologic diseases, seizures at onset • Respiratory distress	• Physical examination findings similar to those of preeclampsia, plus clonic or tonic seizures • Coma or semiconscious state follows convulsions; also, hypertension, increased respiration, cyanosis, fever, pronounced proteinuria, oliguria, pronounced edema • After delivery, urinary output increases and edema diminishes; blood pressure returns to normal within 2 weeks • In terminal stage of fatal eclampsia, pulmonary edema, cyanosis, and other signs of heart failure
Placenta previa • Higher incidence in women over age 35 and in multiparas; tendency for recurrence • A scar on lower uterus, such as from a previous cesarean section • History of placenta previa • An enlarged placenta due to fetal erythroblastosis or multiple gestation • Bleeding usually occurs after 24 weeks • Signs and symptoms include sudden, painless, bright red vaginal bleeding.	• Maternal hypotension and fetal bradycardia or tachycardia • Soft, nontender, noncontracting uterus • Possibly an abnormal (oblique or transverse) fetal position • May have large placenta as seen with multiple fetuses or in patient with diabetes • Placental souffle, audible above symphysis pubis with ultrasound monitoring • Diagnostic studies include sonography and placental localization

Continued

Pregnancy Disorders
Continued

HISTORY AND CHIEF COMPLAINTS	PHYSICAL EXAMINATION AND DIAGNOSTIC STUDIES
Abruptio placentae (mild, moderate, or severe) • Most commonly occurs after 20 weeks • Higher incidence in women over age 35 • Predisposing factors include high parity, previous abruptio placentae, hypertension, inferior vena cava compression, folic acid deficiency, abdominal trauma, sudden uterine compression, short umbilical cord • Signs and symptoms include mild to moderate abdominal pain and vaginal bleeding	• In mild to moderate cases, minimal to moderate bleeding, uterine tenderness, moderate abdominal pain, uterine irritability, hypotension • In severe cases, little or no bleeding; uterus hard, like wood; possibly maternal shock; severe, tearing abdominal pain; oliguria; anuria; absence of fetal heart sounds • Diagnostic studies include hemoconcentration, clotting studies, and sonography
Hydatidiform mole • Highest incidence in women over age 45 • Predisposing factors include previous mole and low-protein diet • Signs and symptoms include excessive nausea and vomiting and uterine bleeding (from spotting to profuse hemorrhage)	• Signs usually apparent by 18 weeks; ovaries tender to palpation; tender uterus due to stretching; uterus large for gestational date; rusty drainage; preeclampsia signs may appear before the 20th week; hypertension; fluid retention; proteinuria • Slight drop in RBC count, hemoglobin, and hematocrit • High or rising titers of human chorionic gonadotropin and thyroxine • Increased WBC count • Mole can be identified with ultrasound by third month.

OTHER BODY SYSTEM DISORDERS

Continued

Pregnancy Disorders
Continued

HISTORY AND CHIEF COMPLAINTS	PHYSICAL EXAMINATION AND DIAGNOSTIC STUDIES
Spontaneous abortion (threatened, inevitable, complete, incomplete, missed, habitual) • Usually occurs around 12th week or not later than 20th week • Signs and symptoms include cramps, backache, vaginal bleeding; patient may complain of "not feeling pregnant anymore"; sudden gush of fluid from vagina occurs in inevitable abortion	• Weight loss; abnormally small uterus for gestational age; may find incompetent cervix if repeated abortions have occurred, especially in midpregnancy; abnormal fetal development found in high percentage of spontaneous abortions; negative or ambiguous pregnancy test
Ectopic pregnancy • History of endosalpingitis, adhesions in the fallopian tubes, or uterine or adnexal mass • Signs and symptoms include lower abdominal pain (may be stabbing, sharp, or dull; unilateral or bilateral; constant or intermittent), nausea; vomiting; amenorrhea in about 75% of patients; vaginal spotting or bleeding possible in tubal pregnancy	• Possibly increased pulse rate or decreased blood pressure • Inspection of the umbilicus in a slender woman or one who has an umbilical hernia may reveal Cullen's sign (a blue discoloration due to extensive intraperitoneal hemorrhage) • Pelvic examination may reveal an abnormal pelvic mass • Elevated erythrocyte sedimentation rate • WBC count: 15,000; RBC count: low, with bleeding • Pregnancy test may be negative • Laparoscopy can detect ectopic pregnancy • Culdoscopy can detect an aborted conceptus and clotted blood • Laparotomy confirms the diagnosis

What Happens in Placenta Previa

Placenta previa's the most common cause of bleeding during the last months of pregnancy. It happens when the placenta develops in the lowest part of the uterus, on or near the cervical opening.

Placenta previa's exact cause isn't known, but certain factors may increase a pregnant patient's risk: age 35 or older; high parity; a scar on the lower uterus, such as from a previous cesarean section; a history of placenta previa; an enlarged placenta due to fetal erythroblastosis or multiple gestation.

These factors may contribute to defective vascularization of the decidua basalis in the fundus. This forces the placenta to spread over a wider area in the lower uterine segment to provide an adequate fetal blood supply, so that it approaches or covers the cervical os.

In the last weeks of pregnancy, when the lower uterus contracts and the cervix dilates, placenta previa causes the placental villi to tear away from the uterine wall, exposing the uterine sinuses. Depending on the number of sinuses exposed, bleeding will be profuse, scanty, or nonexistent until labor begins.

If placenta previa isn't detected in time, and if the child isn't delivered, severe maternal bleeding and shock may occur, together with fetal hypoxia and death.

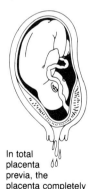

In total placenta previa, the placenta completely covers the os.

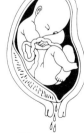

In partial placenta previa, the placenta partially covers the os.

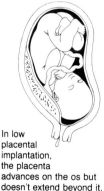

In low placental implantation, the placenta advances on the os but doesn't extend beyond it.

Guide to Urinary Disorders

DISORDER	CHIEF COMPLAINTS
Polycystic kidney disease	• *Output changes:* polyuria • *Voiding pattern changes:* nocturia possible • *Urine color changes:* hematuria, possibly gross • *Pain:* flank pain
Acute pyelonephritis	• *Output changes:* polyuria or none • *Voiding changes:* frequency, urgency • *Urine color changes:* hematuria • *Pain:* tenderness over one or both kidneys
Chronic interstitial nephritis	• *Output changes:* polyuria • *Voiding pattern changes:* nocturia • *Urine color changes:* light color • *Pain:* none
Nephrolithiasis	• *Output changes:* none • *Voiding pattern changes:* frequency, urgency • *Urine color changes:* hematuria • *Pain:* severe, radiating pain
Acute glomerulonephritis	• *Output changes:* oliguria, possibly progressing to anuria • *Voiding pattern changes:* none • *Urine color changes:* hematuria, smoky or coffee-colored • *Pain:* none

HISTORY	EXAMINATION AND DIAGNOSTICS
• Family history of polycystic disease • Symptoms start after age 40	• Enlarged, palpable kidneys • Hypertension • Urine analysis reveals proteinuria, bacteriuria, and calculi. • Further diagnostic studies include urography, ultrasonography, radioisotopic renal scan, renal computerized tomography.
• Sudden onset	• Fever and chills • Nausea and vomiting • Kidneys tender on palpation • Pyuria and bacteriuria
• Urinary abnormality • Early stages may have no specific symptoms.	• Hypertension • Blood analysis reveals elevated BUN. • Urine analysis reveals WBC casts. • Further diagnostic studies include intravenous pyelography and biopsy.
• Excessive dehydration and infection • Previous kidney stones • Hyperparathyroidism • Renal tubular acidosis	• Fever and chills • Nausea and vomiting • Blood analysis reveals leukocytosis. • Urine analysis reveals increased specific gravity, crystalluria, and leukocyturia. • Further diagnostic studies include retrograde intravenous pyelography.
• Poststreptococcal infection of throat or skin • Systemic lupus erythematosus, Schönlein-Henoch purpura, pregnancy, vasculitis, or scleroderma	• Hypertension • Edema • Costovertebral tenderness • Urine analysis reveals proteinuria and RBC casts. • Further diagnostic studies include renal computerized tomography and biopsy.

Continued

Guide to Urinary Disorders
Continued

DISORDER	CHIEF COMPLAINTS
Chronic glomerulone-phritis	• *Output changes:* none • *Voiding pattern changes:* none • *Urine color changes:* none • *Pain:* none
Acute renal artery occlusion	• *Output changes:* oliguria possible • *Voiding pattern changes:* none • *Urine color changes:* none • *Pain:* sudden, sharp, constant pain over upper abdomen or flank
Chronic renal artery stenosis	• *Output changes:* none • *Voiding pattern changes:* none • *Urine color changes:* none • *Pain:* none
Renal vein thrombosis	• *Output changes:* oliguria possible if thrombosis is bilateral • *Voiding pattern changes:* none • *Urine color changes:* hematuria • *Pain:* severe lumbar pain
Acute tubular necrosis	• *Output changes:* oliguria dominates in early stages; leads to renal failure • *Voiding pattern changes:* none • *Urine color changes:* dark and smoky or clear • *Pain:* none

OTHER BODY SYSTEM DISORDERS

HISTORY	EXAMINATION AND DIAGNOSTICS
• May be asymptomatic until advanced stages	• Renal failure • Hypertension • Urine analysis reveals proteinuria. • Blood analysis reveals anemia. • Further diagnostic studies include biopsy.
• Emboli from endocarditis or atherosclerosis	• Severe hypertension • Further diagnostic studies include renal arteriography.
• Fibromuscular dysplasia or atherosclerosis	• Hypertension that's difficult to control • Renal arteriography
• Metastatic disease, nephrotic syndrome, thrombophlebitis, periarteritis, abdominal injury, unexplained leg edema, or recurrent emboli	• Enlargement of affected kidney • Blood analysis reveals leukocytosis. • Urine analysis reveals proteinuria and RBC casts. • Further diagnostic studies include interior venacavography.
• Crush injury or illness associated with shock, such as burns or trauma • Muscle necrosis • Use of a nephrotoxic agent, such as lead or intravenous pyelography dye	• Anorexia • Vomiting • Pulmonary edema, heart failure • Urine analysis reveals low specific gravity, granular casts, and hematuria. • Elevated BUN and creatinine levels • Further diagnostic studies include spot urine sodium and urine creatinine analyses.

Continued

OTHER BODY SYSTEM DISORDERS

Guide to Urinary Disorders
Continued

DISORDER	CHIEF COMPLAINTS
Carcinoma of the bladder	• *Output changes:* oliguria possible, depending on mass size • *Voiding pattern changes:* frequency, urgency, nocturia • *Urine color changes:* hematuria, intermittent or constant • *Pain:* dysuria, flank pain
Cystitis	• *Output changes:* none • *Voiding pattern changes:* frequency, urgency, nocturia • *Urine color changes:* cloudy, hematuria • *Pain:* dysuria, low back pain, or flank pain
Urethral obstruction	• *Output changes:* may progress to anuria • *Voiding pattern changes:* insufficient bladder emptying; frequency; overflow incontinence • *Urine color changes:* none • *Pain:* bladder spasms
Urethritis	• *Output changes:* polyuria may result from forced fluids • *Voiding pattern changes:* frequency, urgency • *Urine color changes:* hematuria • *Pain:* dysuria possible; burning at start of urination; urethral pain

HISTORY	EXAMINATION AND DIAGNOSTICS
• Exposure to analine dyes • Chronic infestation with schistosomes • Heavy cigarette smoking	• Fever • Flank tenderness, muscle weakness • Blood analysis reveals elevated WBC count and anemia. • Positive urine cytology • Further diagnostic studies include cystography, cystoscopy, and biopsy.
• Recurrent urinary tract infections • Recent chemotherapy, systemic antibiotic therapy • Recent vigorous sexual activity • Commonly affects women	• Suprapubic pain on palpation • Fever • Nausea and vomiting • Inflamed genital area • Urine analysis reveals bacteriuria (10^5/ml). • Urine culture and sensitivity tests repeated 2 weeks after therapy ends.
• Prostatic hypertrophy • Meatal stenosis	• Distended bladder • Rectal exam to check for enlarged prostate in males • Enlarged kidney (to compensate for obstruction) • Further studies include catheterization, KUB radiography or CT scan.
• Infections • Exposure to chemicals or bubble bath • Recent vigorous sexual activity	• Fever • Edema and redness around urinary meatus and vulva • Urethral and/or vaginal discharge

OTHER BODY SYSTEM DISORDERS

Guide to Endocrine Disorders

DEFICIENT HORMONE SECRETION	CHIEF COMPLAINTS
Pituitary tumor	• *Abnormalities of sexual maturity or function:* decreased libido; amenorrhea; impotence; changes in amount of sexual hair (such as beard and pubic) • *Mental status changes:* in advanced stages, drowsiness, stupor, convulsions, mental aberrations
Hypopituitarism	• *Fatigue/weakness:* lethargy; easy fatigability • *Weight changes:* may occur (usually loss) • *Abnormalities of sexual maturity or function:* general loss of secondary sex characteristics; amenorrhea • *Mental status changes:* somnolence, coma
Diabetes insipidus	• *Fatigue/weakness:* may be present • *Weight changes:* weight loss; anorexia • *Mental status changes:* irritability; apathy • *Polyuria/polydipsia:* present, may be severe; nocturia; preference for cold drinks
Hypothyroidism	• *Fatigue/weakness:* present, accompanied by lethargy • *Weight changes:* weight gain • *Abnormalities of sexual maturity or function:* diminished sexual functioning; menorrhagia; impotence • *Mental status changes:* abnormal tranquility; answers to questions inappropriate; slowing of cognitive ability; depression

HISTORY	PHYSICAL EXAMINATION AND DIAGNOSTIC STUDIES
• Neurologic symptoms	• Visual field and visual acuity defects, skin changes, headache, intolerance to cold, increased intracranial pressure • Diagnostic studies include skull X-rays, computerized tomography, and carotid angiography.
• Predisposing factors include congenital abnormalities, acute infections, vascular problems, and pituitary tumor.	• Skin changes, slow pulse rate, hypotension, decreased growth, genital atrophy, loss of teeth, brittle nails, anorexia, constipation • Diagnostic studies include CBC, serum thyroxine, serum triiodothyronine, and urine 17-ketogenic steroids.
• Onset may be insidious or sudden. • Predisposing factors include fright and head injury or tumors.	• Dry skin, poor turgor, headache • Diagnostic studies include plasma osmolality and dehydration tests.
• Predisposing factors include surgery or use of radioiodine to treat hyperthyroidism. • Onset usually insidious.	• Sparse, brittle, coarse hair; muscle stiffness; diminished hearing; sensitivity to cold; constipation; hoarseness • Diagnostic studies include serum thyroxine, serum triiodothyronine, and basal metabolic rates.

OTHER BODY SYSTEM DISORDERS

Continued

Guide to Endocrine Disorders
Continued

DEFICIENT HORMONE SECRETION	CHIEF COMPLAINTS
Myxedema (severe Hypothyroidism)	• *Fatigue/weakness:* present, accompanied by lethargy; need for increased amount of sleep • *Weight changes:* weight gain, decreased appetite • *Abnormalities of sexual maturity or function:* diminished sexual functioning, menorrhagia, impotence • *Mental status changes:* in extreme cases, coma, overt psychosis possible
Multinodal goiter	• Usual chief complaints of endocrine disorders not present
Addison's disease (primary adrenal insufficiency)	• *Fatigue/weakness:* slow, progressing fatigue and weakness • *Weight changes:* weight loss caused by poor appetite, food idiosyncrasies, nausea, vomiting, diarrhea • *Abnormalities of sexual maturity or function:* loss of secondary sex characteristics and libido in females • *Mental status changes:* depression, irritability, restlessness

HISTORY	PHYSICAL EXAMINATION AND DIAGNOSTIC STUDIES
• Predisposing factors include long-standing hypothyroidism, exposure to cold, use of respiratory depressants, such as anesthetics.	• Hypothyroidism symptoms continue. • Dry, scaling, cool, yellow-orange, thickened skin; dull, expressionless face; hypothermia; heart enlarged, rate lowered; edema, especially periorbital; thickened tongue; decreased deep tendon reflexes • Diagnostic studies include serum thyroxine, serum triiodothyronine, and basal metabolic rates.
• More common in women • Patient may be asymptomatic for years. • Predisposing factors include iodine deficiency, familial history of disorder.	• Tenderness and visible enlargement of neck; respiratory difficulty, stridor, sensation of choking, hoarseness • Diagnostic studies include serum thyroxine and ^{123}I.
• Onset is insidious. • Predisposing factors include history of tuberculosis, treatment with exogenous steroids, and family history of adrenal insufficiency.	• Fasting hypoglycemia • Hypotension and syncope • Poor coordination • Blue-gray hyperpigmentation on exposed areas of body and mucous membranes, occasionally with vitiligo • Abdominal pain • Salt craving from hyponatremia • Diagnostic studies include plasma cortisol and urine 17-ketogenic steroids.

Continued

Guide to Endocrine Disorders
Continued

DEFICIENT HORMONE SECRETION	CHIEF COMPLAINTS
Diabetes mellitus	• *Fatigue/weakness:* fatigue possible; loss of strength • *Weight changes:* weight loss; in chronic illness, bloating, fullness • *Abnormalities of sexual maturity or function:* impotence in males • *Polyuria/polydipsia:* present; classic symptoms of diabetes mellitus
Hypoparathyroidism	• *Fatigue/weakness:* lethargy • *Mental status changes:* irritability, emotional lability, impaired memory, confusion, depression, changes in level of consciousness, delayed relaxation phase of deep tendon reflexes • *Circulatory changes:* bradycardia, decreased pulse pressure, and decreased cardiac output *Peripheral change:* chills; dry, cold skin

HISTORY	PHYSICAL EXAMINATION AND DIAGNOSTIC STUDIES
• Predisposing factors include long-standing obesity, pancreatic disease, history in females of delivering large infants, and family history of diabetes. • In Type II, mild symptoms may be long-standing.	• Dry skin and mucous membranes, polyphagia, blurred vision, light-headedness, pruritus • In chronic illness, intermittent claudication, especially of feet; pain; paresthesia; hyperpigmentation; xanthomas; poor healing; microaneurysms and exudates in eyes; decreased sensation to pain and temperature; lipodystrophy (from repeated insulin injections); gastrointestinal hyperactivity; decreased perspiration; decreased reflexes • Diagnostic studies include fasting blood sugar and glucose tolerance tests. • Plasma insulin test determines if the patient has an insulin deficiency or is insulin-resistant • A glycosylated hemoglobin test reflects the average plasma glucose concentration over the life span (120 days) of the erythrocytes.
• Predisposing factors include injury to or removal of thyroid (parathyroids taken with thyroid).	• Tetany, paresthesias (numbness and tingling in fingers, toes, and around lips), cyanosis; Chvostek's sign, laryngeal stridor, dyspnea; papilledema (sometimes associated with increased intracranial pressure); malformed, pitted nails; thinning hair, alopecia; coarse, dry skin; dysplasia of tooth enamel; diplopia, cataracts, eyes sensitive to light; convulsions, abdominal pain, nausea, vomiting; EKG changes; Parkinson-like symptoms • Diagnostic studies include serum electrolytes, primarily calcium.

OTHER BODY SYSTEM DISORDERS

Continued

Guide to Endocrine Disorders
Continued

EXCESSIVE HORMONE SECRETION	CHIEF COMPLAINTS
Syndrome of inappropriate antidiuretic hormone secretion	• *Fatigue/weakness:* weakness, lethargy • *Weight changes:* weight gain • *Mental status changes:* confusion, possibly progressing to convulsions and coma
Acromegaly	• *Fatigue/weakness:* progressive weakness • *Abnormalities of sexual maturity or function:* in early stages, increased libido, hypertrophy of genitalia; in later stages, decreased libido, galactorrhea, amenorrhea, impotence, deepening voice • *Mental status changes:* emotional instability • *Polyuria/polydipsia:* present
Hyperthyroidism (thyrotoxicosis)	• *Fatigue/weakness:* weakness present and prominent, increased fatigue; muscle atrophy • *Weight changes:* decreased subcutaneous fat; weight loss despite increase in appetite • *Abnormalities of sexual maturity or function:* short and scanty menstrual periods; decreased fertility; possibly temporal recession of hairline in females • *Mental status changes:* anxiety; nervousness; agitation; paranoid tendencies • *Polyuria/polydipsia:* polyuria possible, with increased thirst

HISTORY	PHYSICAL EXAMINATION AND DIAGNOSTIC STUDIES
• Cancer, head injury, meningitis, encephalitis, brain abscess, cerebrovascular accident, neurosurgery to midbrain, tuberculosis.	• Retention of fluids • Diagnostic studies include BUN, serum creatinine, urine sodium, serum osmolality, serum antidiuretic hormone.
• Insidious onset in third decade of life • Patient will report an increase in hat, glove, shoe size after puberty • Rapid growth spurt or growth in adult life	• Face broadened; overgrowth of lips, nose, tongue, jaw, forehead; pain and stiffness in fingers and toes; increased pigmentation of skin; skin creases; sweating; increased facial hair; edema; hypertension; enlarged internal organs: heart, liver, spleen, glands; polyphagia; headache, visual disturbances, paresthesia • Diagnostic studies include X-rays and glucose tolerance test for growth hormone.
• Predisposing factors include recent emotional crisis, infection, physical stress, family history of Graves' disease. • Relatively common disorder; symptoms depend on severity of disorder.	• Fine, moist palmar erythema; thin and brittle hair and nails; palpable thyroid; systolic bruit over thyroid; possibly tender supraclavicular lymph nodes; palpitations, tachycardia, paroxysmal atrial tachycardia; increased heat production, with excessive perspiration and decreased tolerance to heat; exophthalmos and lid lag characteristic of Graves' disease; pretibial edema; insomnia; fine tremors, exaggerated reflexes • Diagnostic studies include serum thyroxine and serum triiodothyronine.

Continued

Guide to Endocrine Disorders
Continued

EXCESSIVE HORMONE SECRETION	CHIEF COMPLAINTS
Cushing's syndrome	• *Fatigue/weakness:* present, loss of muscle mass • *Weight changes:* weight gain; distribution of fat increases on neck, face, abdomen, girdle • *Abnormalities of sexual maturity or function:* hirsutism, clitoral hypertrophy, amenorrhea in females; gynecomastia in males • *Mental status changes:* irritability, emotional lability, depression, psychosis • *Polyuria/polydipsia:* may be present with other symptoms of diabetes mellitus
Adrenal virilizing syndromes	• *Abnormalities of sexual maturity or function:* reversal of primary and secondary sex characteristics, scanty menstrual periods, amenorrhea, increased sexual drive
Thyroid tumors	• May present with none of the usual chief complaints of thyrotoxicosis or of endocrine disorders

HISTORY	PHYSICAL EXAMINATION AND DIAGNOSTIC STUDIES
• Predisposing factors include steroid treatment and adrenal tumors. • More common in women	• Hypertension; osteoporosis, spontaneous fractures, height reduction, backache, purple striae on arms, breasts, abdomen, and thighs; petechial hemorrhages, excessive bruising; decreased healing ability • Diagnostic studies include serum electrolytes, plasma cortisol, and urine 17-hydroxycorticosteroids.
• May be congenital or acquired • More common in women • Difficult to detect in postpubertal males • Congenital syndromes are believed to be caused by mutant autosomal recessive genes.	• Hirsutism of face, body, and extremities in females; thinning of hair, temporal baldness in males; deepening of voice, Adam's apple enlargement; acne, increased sebum production; development of male habitus, increased muscle mass and increased strength; breast and uterus atrophy, enlargement of clitoris • Diagnostic studies include 17-ketosteroids and 17-hydroxycorticosteroids in urine; dexamethasone suppression test; testosterone levels; adrenal tomography and adrenal angiography.
• Predisposing factors include radiation for thymic enlargement and congenital metabolic defects	• Hoarseness; pain in neck area, difficulty swallowing; enlarged cervical lymph nodes • In thyrotoxicosis, tachycardia, heart failure, vascular collapse, hyperthermia • Diagnostic studies include ^{123}I scan, biopsy, serum thyroxine, and serum triiodothyronine.

OTHER BODY SYSTEM DISORDERS

Continued

Guide to Endocrine Disorders
Continued

EXCESSIVE HORMONE SECRETION	CHIEF COMPLAINTS
Pheochromocytomas (tumor of adrenal medulla)	• *Fatigue/weakness:* malaise • *Weight changes:* weight loss • *Mental status changes:* nervousness; apprehension; feelings of impending doom (prodrome of attack)
Primary aldosteronism	• *Fatigue/weakness:* muscle weakness; fatigue • *Polyuria/polydipsia:* polyuria present; polydipsia possible
Fasting hypoglycemia	• *Fatigue/weakness:* lethargy, weakness, paralysis • *Weight changes:* weight gain • *Mental status changes:* inability to concentrate; changes in sensorium; irritability; inappropriate affect
Hyperparathyroidism	• *Fatigue/weakness:* weakness, fatigability • *Weight changes:* weight loss, anorexia • *Mental status changes:* difficulty concentrating; disorientation; delirium; psychosis; confusion, stupor; coma • *Polyuria/polydipsia:* polyuria may cause polydipsia

HISTORY	PHYSICAL EXAMINATION AND DIAGNOSTIC STUDIES
• Familial incidence most common between ages 40 and 60 • Sudden emotion or physical changes may precipitate attack.	• Hypertension, dyspnea, paresthesias, tetany, blurred vision, severe and throbbing headache, palpitations (possibly intense), profuse sweating, nausea, vomiting, anorexia, abdominal pain, pallor
• Most common in women between ages 30 and 50 • Predisposing factors include use of oral contraceptives.	• Hypertension, headache, ventricular enlargement, cardiac dysrhythmias, hypokalemia • Diagnostic studies include serum electrolytes and urine 17-hydroxycorticosteroids.
• Predisposing factors include liver disease, family history of diabetes mellitus, and use of alcohol, propranolol, and salicylate. • Most common between ages 40 and 60	• Tachycardia, trembling, blurred vision, pallor, paresthesias, palpitations, sweating, decreased coordination, nausea, vomiting, headache • May lead to seizures • Diagnostic studies include glucose tolerance and fasting blood sugar tests.
• May vary in degree from asymptomatic, insidious onset to rapid onset with severe symptoms • Chronic renal disease • Rickets • Osteomalacia may lead to compensatory hyperparathyroidism.	• Cardiac irregularities; anemia; enlarged head; pathologic fractures; hypotonia of muscles; altered reflexes; decreased hearing; ataxic gait; renal symptoms, such as urinary tract infections, pyelonephritis, renal colic; severe headache; bone pain; epigastric pain; nausea; vomiting; pancreatitis; hoarseness; paresthesias for vibration • Diagnostic studies include serum electrolytes and radioimmunoassay for parathyroid hormone.

Differences Between Juvenile-Onset and Adult-Onset Diabetes

	JUVENILE TYPE	ADULT TYPE
Type of onset	Abrupt	Gradual
Symptoms	Thirst, urinary frequency, increased appetite, weight loss	Sometimes none
Stability	Wide fluctuations of blood sugar with marked sensitivity to diet, exercise, and insulin	Usually easily controlled if patient adheres to a proper diet
Ketoacidosis	Frequent only if therapy is inadequate	Uncommon except with severe stress or infection
Hypoglycemia	More frequent	Uncommon
Control of diabetes	Difficult	Less difficult
Endogenous insulin	Absent	Present
Complications	May occur	May occur
Diet	Most important	Most important
Insulin	Needed by all	Needed by 20% to 30%
Oral hypoglycemia agent	Not indicated	Useful for about 40%

Guide to Life-Threatening Diabetic Complications

COMPLICATIONS	SYMPTOMS	CAUSES
Diabetic ketoacidosis (DKA)	• Anorexia, nausea, vomiting, polyuria, weakness, malaise, Kussmaul's respirations, abdominal pain, hyperglycemia (blood sugar from 400 to 800 mg/100 ml); if untreated, may lead to drowsiness, stupor, coma	• Cessation of insulin, or physical or emotional stress • Occurs predominantly in Type I diabetes (insulin-dependent)
Hyperglycemic hyperosmolar nonketotic coma (HHNC)	• Vomiting, diarrhea, tachycardia, rapid breathing, volume depletion, focal motor seizures, transient hemiplegia, severe hyperglycemia (blood sugar about 1,000 mg/100 ml), possibly leading to stupor and coma	• Stress, burns, steroids, diuretics • Severe dehydration from sustained hyperglycemic diuresis in which patient cannot sustain adequate fluid levels • Occurs predominantly in Type II diabetes (non-insulin-dependent)
Insulin shock (hypoglycemia)	• Sweating; tremors; increased blood pressure, pulse rate, respirations; headache; confusion; incoordination; blood sugar 50 mg/100 ml or less; can lead to seizures, coma	• Too much insulin, too little food, excessive physical activity

OTHER BODY SYSTEM DISORDERS

Reactive Hypoglycemia

Hypoglycemia is an abnormally low glucose level in the bloodstream. It occurs when glucose burns too rapidly; when the glucose release rate falls behind tissue demands; and/or when excessive insulin enters the bloodstream.

Hypoglycemia may be classified in two ways: reactive (functional) hypoglycemia and fasting (spontaneous) hypoglycemia. Reactive hypoglycemia may take several forms. In a diabetic patient, it may result from administration of too much insulin or—less commonly—too much oral hypoglycemia medication. In a mildly diabetic patient (or one in the early stages of diabetes mellitus), reactive hypoglycemia may result from delayed and excessive insulin production after carbohydrate ingestion. Similarly, a nondiabetic patient may suffer reactive hypoglycemia from a sharp increase in insulin output after a meal. Sometimes called postprandial hypoglycemia, this type of reactive hypoglycemia usually disappears when the patient eats something sweet. Postprandial hypoglycemia may also develop after gastrointestinal surgery, such as partial gastrectomy, gastroenterostomy, or pyloroplasty.

Signs and symptoms of reactive hypoglycemia include fatigue and malaise, nervousness, irritability, trembling, tension, headaches, hunger, cold sweats, and rapid heart rate.

Two-Hour Postprandial: Preferred Screening Test

Because the 2-hour postprandial test is a simpler procedure than the oral glucose tolerance test or the fasting plasma glucose test, it's often the preferred test for diabetes screening in patients with any of the following conditions:
• obesity
• family histories of diabetes
• transient glycosuria or hyperglycemia (especially during pregnancy, surgery, or administration of adrenal steroids), or after trauma, emotional stress, myocardial infarction, or cerebrovascular accident
• unexplained hypoglycemia, neuropathy, retinopathy, nephropathy, or peripheral vascular disease
• pregnancy resulting in abortion, premature labor, stillbirth, neonatal death, or an unusually large infant
• recurrent infection, especially boils and abscesses.

Identifying Signs and Symptoms of DIC

When assessing your patient's signs and symptoms, keep in mind that disseminated intravascular coagulation (DIC) is a paradoxic condition that's characterized by abnormal bleeding *and* blood clotting. Certain symptoms you observe (such as restlessness, lethargy, or confusion) may be difficult to classify. But others can be categorized according to the type of abnormalities they reflect. Use the chart below to help you recognize signs and symptoms of DIC.

BLEEDING PROBLEMS

Signs and symptoms
• Abnormal or prolonged bleeding from venipuncture sites, drainage tubes, suture lines; or from the rectum, ears, nose, or other body orifices

• Hemoptysis

• Bloody urine or occult blood in stool

• Bleeding around indwelling (Foley) catheters

• Changes in vital signs, possibly indicating internal bleeding

• Increasing abdominal girth, possibly indicating gastrointestinal bleeding

• Petechiae or ecchymosis

• Vision changes or spots in the patient's field of vision from intraocular bleeding

• In a woman, excessive menstrual bleeding and bleeding from vaginal mucous membranes

CLOTTING PROBLEMS

Signs and symptoms
• Cool, mottled skin

• Absent popliteal, posterior tibial, or pedal pulses

• Cyanosis of fingers, toes, earlobes, or the tip of the nose (possibly leading to necrosis)

• Calf swelling and pain on dorsiflexion

• Cerebral vascular accident

• Renal failure

• Pulmonary embolism

Disseminated Intravascular Coagulation (DIC)

In a patient suffering from DIC, normal clotting accelerates, producing clots in the capillary bed where they are not needed. As a result, clotting factors (fibrinogen, prothrombin, Factor V, Factor VIII, and platelets) are depleted.

Because of this depletion, clots can't form where they're needed. But before the body can replace these now-missing clotting factors, clot-dissolving mechanisms begin dissolving even stable clots. The result is an overabundance of anticoagulant factors, which triggers uncontrolled hemorrhaging.

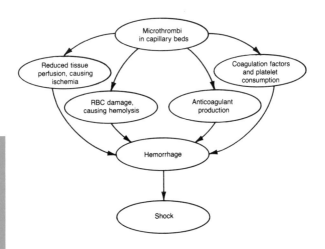

Precipitating Causes of DIC

OBSTETRIC
Abruptio placentae
Retained dead fetus
Amniotic fluid embolism
Retained placenta
Toxemia
HEMOLYTIC
Transfusion of mismatched blood
Acute hemolysis from infection or immunologic disorders
NECROTIC
Extensive burns and trauma
Rejection of transplants
Postoperative necrosis; especially following extracorporeal circulation
NEOPLASTIC
Prostatic cancer
Acute leukemias

Giant cavernous hemangioma
Carcinoma
Sarcoma
INFECTIOUS
Acute bacteria
Virus
Fungus
Protozoa
Rickettsia
MISCELLANEOUS
Fat embolism
Snake bites
Glomerulonephritis
Thrombotic thrombocytopenia purpura
Cirrhosis
Hypotension
Lung surgery
Heatstroke

Managing DIC: Some Nursing Considerations

In addition to identifying early signs and symptoms, your role in DIC management involves correcting the underlying disorders, compensating for anemia and hypovolemia, and preventing additional bleeding. Follow these guidelines:

• Carefully check your patient's blood study results, especially hemoglobin and hematocrit values and coagulation times.

• Give replacement blood or blood products, as ordered, to replace depleted clotting factors and platelets. Watch for transfusion reactions and fluid overload.

• Assist with mechanical ventilation, peritoneal dialysis, or hemodialysis, as ordered.

• Administer oxygen, as ordered.

• To determine your patient's blood loss, weigh the dressings and linen and record the amount of drainage. *Note:* Don't forget to include blood specimens when you document blood loss.

Continued

Managing DIC: Some Nursing Considerations
Continued

• Weigh the patient at the same time each day in the same or similar clothing to check his fluid balance, particularly if he has a kidney disorder. In acute DIC, monitor intake and output hourly.

• Watch for bleeding from the gastrointestinal and genitourinary tracts. If you suspect intraabdominal hemorrhage, measure the patient's abdominal girth every 4 hours. Test specimens of gastric secretions, stool, and urine for blood.

• Be alert for signs and symptoms of hypovolemic shock.

• Check I.V. sites frequently for bleeding.

• Limit intramuscular and subcutaneous injections. Apply pressure to injection site for at least 10 minutes to control the bleeding.

• To prevent blood clots from dislodging and causing fresh bleeding, don't scrub bleeding areas.

• Use pressure, cold compresses, and topical hemostatic agents, such as an absorbable gelatin sponge (Gelfoam), to control the bleeding.

• If ordered, give your patient heparin. *Note:* Heparin therapy to treat DIC is controversial, because heparin disrupts the clotting cascade. Heparin is contraindicated if the patient has brain damage or dysfunction, or if he has a necrotizing lesion.

• If ordered, give your patient aminocaproic acid (Amicar*), an antifibrinolytic agent. Because this drug may cause clots in vital organs, giving it is also controversial.

• Protect your patient from injury. Enforce bed rest and pad the bed's side rails if your patient is agitated.

• Tell co-workers of the patient's tendency to hemorrhage.

• Provide gentle mouth care. Remember, your patient's gums may bleed easily.

• Avoid using adhesive tape. The force needed to remove it may cause bleeding.

• To help control pain from tissue ischemia, administer analgesics that don't contain aspirin, as ordered.

• Perform passive range-of-motion exercises on your patient during nonbleeding periods to reduce joint and muscle pain. Avoid giving back rubs or skin massages because these may promote bleeding.

• Because DIC may cause hemorrhaging in major organs, watch your patient for signs and symptoms of cerebral, gastrointestinal, and hepatic hemorrhage.

• Document all patient care.

*Available in the United States and Canada

Recognizing Transfusion Reactions

If your patient develops any of the following signs or symptoms during a blood transfusion, immediately follow your hospital's procedure for stopping the transfusion and prepare for further treatment.

HEMOLYTIC
Signs and symptoms
Include chills, fever, low back pain, headache, chest pain, tachycardia, dyspnea, hypotension, nausea and vomiting, restlessness, anxiety, shock
Nursing considerations
• Place the patient in a supine position with his legs elevated 20° to 30°, and administer oxygen, fluids, and epinephrine.
• Administer mannitol.
• Insert an indwelling catheter.
• Administer antipyretics. If the patient's fever persists, apply a hypothermia blanket or give tepid sponge or alcohol baths.

PLASMA PROTEIN INCOMPATIBILITY
Signs and symptoms
Include chills, fever, flushing, abdominal pain, diarrhea, dyspnea, hypotension
Nursing considerations
• Place the patient in a supine position with his legs elevated 20° to 30°, and administer oxygen, fluids, and epinephrine.
• Administer corticosteroids.

BLOOD CONTAMINATION
Signs and symptoms
Include chills, fever, abdominal sea and vomiting, bloody diarrhea, hypotension
Nursing considerations
• Administer fluids, antibiotics, corticosteroids, vasopressors, and a fresh transfusion.

FEBRILE
Signs and symptoms
Range from mild chills, flushing, and fever to extreme signs and symptoms resembling a hemolytic reaction
Nursing considerations
• Administer an antipyretic and an antihistamine for a *mild* reaction.
• Treat a *severe* reaction the same as a hemolytic reaction.

ALLERGIC
Signs and symptoms
• Range from pruritus, urticaria, hives, facial swelling, chills, fever, nausea and vomiting, headache, and wheezing to laryngeal edema, respiratory distress, and shock
Nursing considerations
• Administer parenteral antihistamines or, for a severe reaction, epinephrine or corticosteroids.
• If the patient's only sign of reaction is hives, expect to restart the infusion, as ordered, at a slower rate.

Types of Immune Disorders

TYPE/DESCRIPTION	EXAMPLE
Immunodeficiency Deficiency in phagocytosis, immunoglobulin production, cellular functioning, or a combination of these	• *Primary:* DiGeorge's syndrome • *Secondary:* immunosuppression caused by radiation or chemotherapy
Gammopathy Abnormal production of high levels of dysfunctional gamma globulins	• Multiple myeloma, macroglobulinemia
Hypersensitivity (allergy) Exaggerated or inappropriate response to sensitizing antigens, classified as follows:	
Type I (anaphylactic): humoral mediation (IgE binds to mast cells); immediate onset	• Hay fever, allergic asthma, anaphylactic shock
Type II (cytotoxic): humoral mediation (IgG or IgM binds to cell surface antigen); immediate onset	• Transfusion reactions
Type III (immune complex): humoral mediation (IgG or IgM forms complex with soluble antigen); immediate onset	• Serum sickness, acute glomerulonephritis
Type IV (cell-mediated): cellular mediation (T cells and macrophages cause tissue destruction); delayed onset	• Graft rejection, reaction to tubercle bacillus
Autoimmunity Altered discrimination between self and nonself, causing immunologic attack on self antigens	• Pernicious anemia, systemic lupus erythematosus, rheumatoid arthritis, myasthenia gravis

OTHER BODY SYSTEM DISORDERS

Tests for Blood Composition, Production, and Function

Overall composition

• *Peripheral blood smear* shows maturity and morphologic characteristics of blood elements and determines qualitative abnormalities.

• *Complete blood count (CBC)* determines the actual number of blood elements in relation to volume and quantifies abnormalities.

• *Bone marrow aspiration* or *biopsy* allows evaluation of hematopoiesis by showing blood elements and precursors, and abnormal or malignant cells.

RBC function

• *Hematocrit (HCT)* (packed cell volume) measures the percentage of RBCs per fluid volume of whole blood.

• *Hemoglobin (Hgb)* measures the amount (grams) of hemoglobin per 100 ml of blood, to determine oxygen-carrying capacity.

• *Reticulocyte count* allows assessment of RBC production by determining concentration of this early erythrocyte precursor.

• *Schilling test* determines absorption of vitamin B_{12} (necessary for erythropoiesis) by measuring excretion of radioactive B_{12} in the urine.

• *Mean corpuscular volume (MCV)* describes the red cell in terms of size.

• *Mean corpuscular hemoglobin (MCH)* determines average amount of hemoglobin per RBC.

• *Mean corpuscular hemoglobin concentration (MCHC)* establishes average hemoglobin concentration in 100 ml of packed RBCs.

• *Serum bilirubin* measures liver function and extravascular RBC hemolysis.

• *Sugar-water test* assesses the susceptibility of RBCs to hemolyze with complement.

• *Direct Coombs' test* demonstrates the presence of IgG antibodies (such as antibodies to Rh factor) and/or complement of circulating RBCs.

Continued

OTHER BODY SYSTEM DISORDERS

Tests for Blood Composition, Production, and Function
Continued

- *Indirect Coombs' test,* a two-step test, detects the presence of IgG antibodies on RBCs in the serum.
- *Sideroblast test* detects stainable iron (available for hemoglobin synthesis) in normoblastic RBCs.

Hemostasis

- *Platelet count* determines number of platelets.
- *Prothrombin time (Quick's test, pro time, PT)* aids evaluation of thrombin generation (extrinsic clotting mechanism).
- *Partial thromboplastin time (PTT)* aids evaluation of the adequacy of plasma-clotting factors (intrinsic clotting mechanism).
- *Thrombin time* detects abnormalities in thrombin fibrinogen reaction.
- *Activated partial thromboplastin time (APTT)* aids assessment of plasma-clotting factors (except factors VII and XIII) in the intrinsic clotting mechanism.

WBC function

- *WBC count, differential* establishes quantity and maturity of WBC elements (neutrophils [called polymorphonuclear granulocytes or bands], basophils, eosinophils, lymphocytes, monocytes).

Plasma

- *Erythrocyte sedimentation rate (ESR)* measures rate of RBCs settling from plasma and may reflect infection.
- *Electrophoresis of serum proteins* determines amount of various serum proteins (classified by mobility in response to an electrical field).
- *Immunoelectrophoresis of serum proteins* separates and classifies serum antibodies (immunoglobulins) through specific antiserums.
- *Fibrinogen (Factor I)* measures this coagulation factor in plasma.

Oxygen Transportation Disorders

IRON DEFICIENCY ANEMIA

Chief complaint
• *Fatigue and weakness:* present; increases with anemia's severity
History
• Predisposing factors include poor nutrition; chronic blood loss from ulcers, gastritis, or excessive menstruation.
• Signs and symptoms include headache, shortness of breath, pica (craving odd things to eat, such as starch or clay).
• Most common in children, female adolescents, and women in their reproductive years
Physical examination and diagnostic studies
• Tachycardia, functional systolic murmur, slight cardiac and liver enlargement, spoon-shaped nails, poor skin turgor, stomatitis, pallor, ankle edema, menstrual disturbances.
• Diagnostic studies include complete blood count, measurement of serum iron level, possibly bone marrow biopsy; guaiac test performed to detect presence of occult blood in stool.

PERNICIOUS ANEMIA

Chief complaint
• *Fatigue and weakness:* present, accompanied by light-headedness
History
• Predisposing factors include immune disorders, positive family history
• Signs and symptoms: gastrointestinal system—digestion disturbances, nausea, vomiting, diarrhea, constipation, anorexia; central nervous system—neuritis, peripheral numbness and paresthesias, impaired coordination and movement, light-headedness, altered vision; cardiovascular system—palpitations, dyspnea, orthopnea
• Insidious onset; progresses slowly
Physical examination and diagnostic studies
• Pallor, slightly icteric skin and eyes, rapid pulse rate, cardiomegaly and possibly systolic murmur, slight hepatosplenomegaly, positive Romberg's sign and Babinski's reflex, altered mental status.
• Diagnostic studies include gastric analysis for decreased acid and pepsin secretion, bone marrow aspiration, complete blood count, assay for serum vitamin B_{12}, Schilling test.

Continued

Oxygen Transportation Disorders
Continued

APLASTIC ANEMIA

Chief complaints
- *Abnormal bleeding:* mild bleeding from nose, gums, vagina, or gastrointestinal tract
- *Fatigue and weakness:* mild and progressive
- *Fever:* may be present

History
- Predisposing factors include use of medication, such as chloramphenicol or benzene derivatives, that suppresses bone marrow; therapeutic X-rays; infectious hepatitis
- Insidious onset

Physical examination and diagnostic studies
- Pallor, ecchymoses, petechiae
- Diagnostic studies include complete blood count, measurement of serum iron level, total iron-binding capacity, bone marrow biopsy.

HEMOLYTIC ANEMIAS

Chief complaint
- *Fatigue and weakness:* present, variable

History
- Predisposing factors include chronic immune-related illness, such as systemic lupus erythematosus; neoplastic disease; recent cardiac trauma; use of such drugs as amphotericin; toxin or poison ingestion; blood transfusion incompatibility; positive family history.

Physical examination and diagnostic studies
- Mild jaundice, pallor
- Orthostatic hypotension, tachycardia, some cardiac murmurs
- Splenomegaly possible
- Diagnostic studies include complete blood count, bone marrow biopsy, Coombs' test, urine test for urobilinogen.

SICKLE CELL ANEMIA

Chief complaints
- *Fatigue and weakness:* may be present
- *Fever:* present
- *Joint pain:* may be severe and involve multiple joints

History
- Recurrent infections caused by increased susceptibility
- Inherited genes from both parents
- Signs and symptoms include dyspnea, aching bones, chest pain.
- Infection, stress, dehydration, and conditions that provoke hypoxia may provoke periodic crisis.
- Most common in blacks of African descent

Continued

Oxygen Transportation Disorders
Continued

SICKLE CELL ANEMIA
Continued

Physical examination and diagnostic studies
• Asthenic habitus with disproportionately long arms and legs in adulthood; retarded growth; delayed sexual maturity; tachycardia, cardiomegaly, and systolic murmurs; pulmonary infarctions; hepatomegaly leading to cirrhosis; jaundice, pallor; joint swelling; ischemic leg ulcers
• Diagnostic studies include hemoglobin electrophoresis, liver biopsy, stained blood smear showing sickle cells, complete blood count.

Cell Proliferation Disorders

PRIMARY POLYCYTHEMIA (polycythemia vera)

Chief complaints
• *Abnormal bleeding:* nosebleeds, spontaneous bruising, bleeding ulcers
• *Fatigue and weakness:* present
• *Joint pain:* may be present
History
• Signs and symptoms include headaches; dizziness; tinnitus, and vertigo; blurred vision; pruritus; chest pain; dyspnea; gastrointestinal distress; intermittent claudication.
• May be asymptomatic in early stages
• Most common in Jewish males from middle to old age
Physical examination and diagnostic studies
• Plethora or ruddy cyanosis of face, hands, and mucous membranes; ecchymoses; engorged conjunctival and retinal veins on ophthalmoscopic examination; enlarged, firm, and nontender spleen; hypertension, thrombosis, or emboli
• Diagnostic studies include complete blood count, bone marrow biopsy, and analysis of arterial blood gases.

ACUTE LEUKEMIA

Chief complaints
• *Abnormal bleeding:* nose and gum bleeding, easy bruising, prolonged menses
• *Lymphadenopathy:* present; may be generalized or primarily involve cervical nodes *Continued*

OTHER BODY SYSTEM DISORDERS

Cell Proliferation Disorders
Continued

ACUTE LEUKEMIA
Continued

• *Fatigue and weakness:* present; severity depends on extent of illness
• *Fever:* may be high- or low-grade
History
• Exposure to radiation or benzene derivatives is a predisposing factor.
• Signs and symptoms include headache, tinnitus, shortness of breath, chills, recurrent infections, abdominal or bone pain.
Physical examination and diagnostic studies
• Petechiae, ecchymoses, pallor, edema, splenomegaly, retinal hemorrhages on ophthalmoscopic examination
• Diagnostic studies include complete blood count with differential and bone marrow aspiration and biopsy.

CHRONIC LEUKEMIA

Chief complaints
• *Abnormal bleeding:* rare
• *Lymphadenopathy:* may be present
• *Fatigue and weakness:* may be present; characterized by vague feeling of malaise and fatigue
• *Fever:* low-grade and unexplained in lymphocytic leukemia

History
• Predisposing factors include exposure to therapeutic or accidental radiation or to such chemicals as benzene or alkalyzing agents.
• Signs and symptoms include anorexia, weight loss, bone tenderness.
Physical examination and diagnostic studies
• Splenomegaly, hepatomegaly, edema, anemia; in lymphocytic leukemia, papular or vesicular skin lesions, herpes zoster, collapsed vertebrae
• Increased white blood cell count with proliferation of one type of white cell
• Further diagnostic studies include complete blood count with differential count and bone marrow aspiration or biopsy.

HODGKIN'S DISEASE

Chief complaints
• *Lymphadenopathy:* asymmetrical enlargement usually involves cervical nodes but occasionally involves axillary or inguinal or femoral nodes
• *Fever:* may be present
History
• Signs and symptoms include generalized and severe pruritus; anorexia and weight loss in advanced stage.

Continued

Cell Proliferation Disorders
Continued

HODGKIN'S DISEASE
Continued

• 50% of cases occur in persons aged 20 to 40.
Physical examination and diagnostic studies
• Enlarged, rubbery, painless nodes; splenomegaly; anemia
• Symptoms depend on nodes affected and disease stage.
• Diagnostic studies include lymphangiography; lymph node, bone marrow, liver, and spleen biopsies; blood tests; chest X-ray; staging laparotomy, gallium scan, ultrasound of abdomen.

MULTIPLE MYELOMA

Chief complaint
• *Abnormal bleeding:* may be present
• *Fatigue and weakness:* present; possibly severe
• *Fever:* present
History
• Signs and symptoms: mild, transient skeletal pain progressing to severe back, rib, or extremity pain; decreased urinary output; anorexia and weight loss; repeated bacterial infections
• Most common in middle-aged and elderly men
Physical examination and diagnostic studies
• Bone deformities
• Anemia, possible hepatosplenomegaly, renal insufficiency, peripheral neuropathy
• Diagnostic studies include CBC, bone marrow aspiration, urine tests for protein and calcium, serum electrophoresis for protein, skeletal survey, intravenous pyelography.

Immune Complex Disorders

SYSTEMIC LUPUS ERYTHEMATOSUS

Chief complaint
• *Abnormal bleeding:* heavy menses possible
• *Lymphadenopathy:* enlargement without tenderness
• *Fatigue and weakness:* present
• *Fever:* present
• *Joint pain:* arthralgia in fingers, hands, wrists, ankles, and knees
History
• Predisposing factors include genetic disorder, viral infections
• Signs and symptoms include weight loss, anorexia, malaise, muscle pain, cough
• Most common in females aged 10 to 35

Continued

Immune Complex Disorders
Continued

SYSTEMIC LUPUS ERYTHEMATOSUS *Continued*

Physical examination and diagnostic studies
• Butterfly rash with blush and swelling or scaly maculopapular rash on cheeks and bridge of nose; pigmentation changes; patchy alopecia; pleural effusion; pericarditis; myocarditis; nephritis; Raynaud's phenomenon; hepatomegaly; convulsive disorders; mental status changes
• Diagnostic studies include antinuclear antibody test, Coombs' test, rheumatoid factor, LE-cell test, skin and renal biopsy.

RHEUMATOID ARTHRITIS

Chief complaint
• *Abnormal bleeding:* easy bruising in long-standing disease
• *Lymphadenopathy:* generalized, or present only in the nodes proximal to the involved peripheral joints
• *Fatigue and weakness:* generalized
• *Fever:* may rise to 100.4° F.
• *Joint pain:* joint stiffness and swelling; in advanced stages, deformities; vague arthralgias and myalgias; limited ROM
History
• Insidious or acute onset

• Most common in women aged 40 to 50
Physical examination and diagnostic studies
• Keratoconjunctivitis sicca; increased warmth, tenderness, and swelling of involved joints; rheumatoid nodules possible; skin ulcers; muscle atrophy; pleural effusion possible
• Diagnostic studies include ESR, latex agglutination test for rheumatoid factor, antinuclear antibody test, synovial fluid analysis, joint X-rays.

SYSTEMIC SCLEROSIS

Chief complaint
• *Abnormal bleeding:* present, in gastrointestinal tract
• *Fatigue and weakness:* vague
• *Fever:* rare, may reflect concurrent problem
• *Joint pain:* diffuse aching and stiffness, polyarticular arthritis; deformities and immobility caused by skin encasement
History
• History of Raynaud's phenomenon
• Signs and symptoms include weight loss and exertional dyspnea, dysphagia, heartburn.
• Most common in women aged 20 to 50

Continued

Immune Complex Disorders
Continued

SYSTEMIC SCLEROSIS
Continued

- Family history rare
- Raynaud's phenomenon; thickened edematous skin that becomes waxy, taut, and atrophic; pigmentation changes; telangiectasias; pulmonary interstitial fibrosis; progressive cardiac involvement; progressive renal failure
- Diagnostic studies include ESR, rheumatoid factor, antinuclear antibody test, skin biopsy, gastrointestinal X-rays, hand X-rays.

POLYMYOSITIS/DERMATO-MYOSITIS

Chief complaint
- *Fatigue and weakness:* insidious onset in proximal muscles of arms and legs
- *Fever:* possibly low-grade, intermittent, appearing after development of muscle weakness
- *Joint pain:* arthralgia
- *Skin changes:* characteristic reddish purple rash with minimal scaling; distribution is predominantly on the face and upper chest, but the rash may develop over prominences such as the hands, elbows, knees, and ankles; heliotrope rash may be present on the upper lids.
- *Dysphagia:* from esophageal weakness

History
- Predisposing factors include respiratory or obscure systemic illnesses, neoplastic lesions, other connective tissue diseases. However, first symptoms may develop during excellent health
- Signs and symptoms include myalgias, dysphagia, anorexia, weight loss, dyspnea, photosensitivity.
- Most common in females aged 5 to 15 and 45 to 60

Physical examination and diagnostic studies
- Raynaud's phenomenon: dusky erythema over face, shoulders, and arms; heliotrope rash over eyelids; scaling maculopapular lesions over bony prominences; contractures
- Diagnostic studies include ESR, CBC, serum enzymes, rheumatoid factor, electromyography, muscle biopsy.
- Results may be elevated for the following laboratory tests: nonspecific hypergammaglobulinemia; antinuclear antibodies and rheumatoid factors; serum enzymes, such as CPK, SGOT, and urine creatinine and myoglobin.

Four Types of Hyperimmunity

Hyperimmune states have been grouped into four major types:

• *Type I* (immediate hypersensitivity): Antigen reacts with a sensitized antibody (IgE) fixed on the surfaces of mast cells or basophils, causing release of vasoactive amines and histamine. These amines produce allergic symptoms, such as hives, secretions, erythema, itching, smooth-muscle contraction, and, possibly, shock.

• *Type II* (cytotoxic): Antibody reacts with an antigenic component of a cell, or with an antigen or a hapten associated with a cell. Complement or moncnuclear cells (lymphocytic macrophages) cause actual cellular destruction, resulting in lysis of the target cell. Thus, if erythrocytes are the target, such destruction causes hemolytic anemia; if platelets are the target, thrombocytopenia; and if white cells are the target, leukopenia.

• *Type III* (immune-complex mediated): Complexes of antigen-antibody and complement, forming in the blood, may precipitate onto "innocent bystander" cells and tissues, which are damaged by local inflammation. Type III hyperimmune conditions include glomerulonephritis, arteritis, and rheumatoid arthritis.

• *Type IV* (delayed hypersensitivity): Sensitized T cells respond to antigens by excessive release of lymphokines or by direct cytotoxic injury. Type IV reactions are a delayed type of sensitivity, requiring 48 to 72 hours for reaction. This form of hypersensitivity includes allergic contact dermatitis, resulting from exposure to poison ivy, and skin reactions to cosmetics.

Clinical Clues to T- or B-Cell Deficiency

T-cell deficiency
• Decreased lymphocyte count with fungal and viral diseases
• Systemic illness after vaccination with live virus or bacille Calmette-Guérin
• Graft-versus-host reaction after blood transfusion, with skin rash, diarrhea, jaundice, and infection
• Low serum calcium levels in newborns with DiGeorge's syndrome

B-cell deficiency
• Decreased serum immunoglobulin levels and recurrent pyogenic infections

Combined T- and B-cell deficiencies
• Decreased lymphocyte count and immunoglobulin levels
• Recurrent pyogenic, viral, or fungal infections

Fracture

Chief complaints
- *Pain:* intensity increases until fragments are set
- *Joint stiffness:* may be present with fracture near joint; crepitation
- *Swelling and redness:* varying degrees of swelling and bleeding into tissues
- *Deformity and immobility:* bone deformity; bone may project through skin; lost or diminished function of fractured part
- *Sensory changes:* Initial trauma, bleeding, and swelling may cause pressure on nerves

History
- Direct trauma
- Indirect trauma above or below injury site
- Predisposing factors include repeated stress, osteogenic sarcoma, osteoporosis, Paget's disease, hematopoietic diseases, nutritional deficiencies.

Physical findings
- Bone contour defect, abnormal bone motion, possibly shock
- Diagnostic studies include X-rays

Do's and Don'ts of Fracture Care

- Do ease your patient's pain and distress by explaining what you're going to do.
- Don't straighten a severely angulated extremity before immobilizing it.
- Don't push protruding bone ends into your patient's skin when you immobilize the injured extremity.
- Do remember to pad the splint before you apply it.
- Don't constrict your patient's circulation when you immobilize his injured part.
- Do check your patient's immobilized extremity every 15 minutes for possible temperature and color changes.
- Do elevate the patient's injured extremity above his heart after you splint it, to decrease risk of edema.
- Do look for signs that your patient may have internal hemorrhaging, increased pain, or shock. For example, stay alert for personality changes, restlessness, or irritability.
- Do give your patient medication for pain, as ordered by the doctor.
- Do notify the doctor if you have problems with your patient's traction device.

Bone Disorders

DISORDER	CHIEF COMPLAINTS
Osteoarthritis	• *Pain:* during inclement weather; worse after exposure to cold, exercise, or weight-bearing; relieved by rest • *Joint stiffness:* transient stiffness worse in morning or after inactivity; affects weight-bearing joints • *Swelling and redness:* joints swollen and tender but not red or hot • *Deformity and immobility:* Heberden's nodes in distal joints; Bouchard's nodes in proximal joints; flexion contracture possible
Gout	• *Pain:* present, severe; worse after high purine food ingestion; frequently nocturnal; onset usually sudden • *Joint stiffness:* joint immobility caused by pain and swelling • *Swelling and redness:* red or cyanotic, tense, hot skin over affected swollen joint; in acute form, usually monoarticular • *Deformity and immobility:* painless tophi (urate deposits) in external ears, hands, elbows, and knees; can't bear weight on affected limb
Reiter's syndrome	• *Pain:* present • *Joint stiffness:* present, usually in sacroiliac joint and sometimes in foot, knee, or ankle joints; weight-bearing joint involvement usually asymmetrical • *Swelling and redness:* signs of acute inflammation • *Deformity and immobility:* presence depends on extent of arthritis that is part of Reiter's syndrome

HISTORY	PHYSICAL EXAMINATION AND DIAGNOSTIC STUDIES
• Onset usually after age 55 • Moderate to severe disease more common in postmenopausal women • Predisposing factors include joint damage from trauma, infection, or stress; dietary calcium deficiency; history of arthritis in one or both parents; occupation.	• Decreased range of motion; altered bone contour; bony enlargement; malaligned joints; no systemic manifestations; crepitation on motion • Diagnostic studies include X-rays of affected joints.
• Predisposing factors include renal disease, family history of gout, disorders that cause alterations in purine metabolism or decreased renal clearance of uric acid.	• Altered bone contour; elevated blood pressure; tachycardia; fever; nephrolithiasis; renal failure; thickened, wrinkled, desquamated skin • Diagnostic studies include uric acid levels, complete blood count; synovial fluid analysis; arthroscopy.
• More common in young men • Recent sexual activity • Cause unknown	• Limited range of motion • Lesions of mucous membranes, oral and genital skin, and nails; resembles psoriasis; lesions with yellow vesicles on soles and palms; low-grade fever; conjunctivitis; urethritis • Diagnostic studies include synovial fluid analysis.

OTHER BODY SYSTEM DISORDERS

Continued

Bone Disorders
Continued

DISORDER	CHIEF COMPLAINTS
Ankylosing spondylitis (Marie-Strümpell disease)	• *Pain:* begins as lower backache that radiates down thighs • *Joint stiffness:* decreased joint mobility and muscle stiffness • *Swelling and redness:* present, resembling rheumatoid arthritis, synovitis • *Deformity and immobility:* progressively limited back movement and chest expansion; in severe cases, fusion of entire spine
Osteomyelitis	• *Pain:* present in affected joint with movement • *Joint stiffness:* restricted movement caused by pain • *Swelling and redness:* onset of swelling in 1 to 2 days; inflammation • *Deformity and immobility:* joint may be immobilized by pain
Osteoporosis	• *Pain:* possible; symptom of fracture or vertebral collapse; aggravated by movement • *Deformity and immobility:* fractures of involved bones; collapse of vertebrae; increasing kyphosis or dowager's hump possible

HISTORY	PHYSICAL EXAMINATION AND DIAGNOSTIC STUDIES
• Most common in male children and young male adults ages 10 to 30 • Familial disorder; genetic predisposition	• Decreased spinal range of motion; abnormal vertebrae alignment; flattened lumbar curve; exaggerated thoracic curvature; decreased chest expansion; cardiac complication with long-standing disease; atrophy of trunk muscles; fever; fatigue; weight loss • Diagnostic studies include X-rays and HLA antigen studies.
• Predisposing factors include recent infection, surgery, fracture, puncture wound, bites, prolonged drug addiction. • Sudden onset	• Limited range of motion; unequal limb circumferences; local necrosis or lesion on skin surface; fever; chills; malaise • Diagnostic studies include blood cultures and X-rays.
• Predisposing factors include endocrine disorders, excessive cigarette smoking, chronic low dietary calcium intake, malabsorption, prolonged immobility. • Most common in postmenopausal women	• Evidence of healed fracture; loss of height; wedging of dorsal vertebrae or anterior vertebrae • Diagnostic studies include X-rays and bone densitometry measurements.

Continued

OTHER BODY SYSTEM DISORDERS

Bone Disorders
Continued

DISORDER	CHIEF COMPLAINTS

Paget's disease

- *Pain:* present in deep bone
- *Joint stiffness:* present, as in rheumatoid arthritis
- *Swelling and redness:* increased heat in affected area from increased vascularity
- *Deformity and immobility:* bowing of long bones; kyphosis; frequent fractures with slight trauma
- *Sensory changes:* headaches, deafness, vertigo, tinnitus, or other sensory changes possible; caused by bony growth that compresses nerves

Osteogenic sarcoma

- *Pain:* persistent and progressive; local at first, then diffuse; bone tenderness
- *Joint stiffness:* if tumor is located in joint
- *Swelling and redness:* present in area of tumor; appears gradually as tumor grows; variable swelling; local heat
- *Deformity and immobility:* pathological fractures; limited movement of affected part

Cervical disk herniation

- *Pain:* present in neck, shoulder, or arm; exact distribution depends on which nerve route is compressed; increases with neck flexion and rotation; paroxysmal
- *Deformity and immobility:* limited neck range of motion; muscle (biceps) weakness
- *Sensory changes:* paresthesia and sensory loss over neck, shoulder, arm, and/or hand, depending on specific nerve root involvement

HISTORY	PHYSICAL EXAMINATION AND DIAGNOSTIC STUDIES
• Predisposing factors include recent deafness, family history of Paget's disease, cardiovascular and pulmonary disease. • More prevalent over age 40 • Most common in men	• Altered bone contour; waddling gait; increased head size • Diagnostic studies include blood tests for increased calcium and alkaline phosphatase; bone scan; X-rays.
• Peak incidence at age 20 • More common in males • Accompanying factors include weight loss. • Predisposing factors include history of Paget's disease, exposure to radiation, trauma.	• Decreased range of motion; unequal limb circumferences; venous engorgement; anemia • Diagnostic studies include biopsy and X-rays.
• Recent neck trauma or forceful hyperextension • May be related to intervertebral joint degeneration	• Cough, sneeze, or strain (downward pressure on head) in hyperextended position causes pain; diminished biceps or triceps jerk • Diagnostic studies include X-rays, myelography, computerized tomography scan.

Continued

OTHER BODY SYSTEM DISORDERS

Bone Disorders
Continued

DISORDER	CHIEF COMPLAINTS
Herniated lumbosacral disk (lower back pain)	• *Pain:* present with coughing, sneezing, straining, bending, or lifting; increases with sitting; occurs over dermatome for that specific disk; accompanied by mild or severe low back, buttock, or leg pain; may be associated with spasms • *Joint stiffness:* inflexible spine • *Deformity and immobility:* muscle atrophy of affected extremities • *Sensory changes:* decreased sensation, paresthesias; absent reflexes over dermatomes; voiding or defecating difficulties, particularly urinary retention
Scoliosis	• *Pain:* present; radiates from back to extremities • *Joint stiffness:* hip or knee flexion contractures • *Deformity and immobility:* rib cage deformity; hamstring tightness; the higher the location of the scoliosis, the more severe the deformity • *Sensory changes:* decreased sensation to lower extremities
Kyphosis	• *Pain:* present in back; radiates to legs • *Joint stiffness:* stiff back • *Deformity and immobility:* round back in thoracic region; lordotic curve; hamstring tightness • *Sensory changes:* decreased sensation in lower legs

HISTORY	PHYSICAL EXAMINATION AND DIAGNOSTIC STUDIES
• Predisposing factors include recent spinal trauma, heavy lifting, or occupational stress on back; lack of exercise; weight gain; degenerative changes.	• Decreased spinal range of motion; unequal limb circumferences; abnormal posture; scoliosis; abnormal leg reflexes; diminished ankle or knee jerk; positive straight-leg–raising test (limited ability to straight-raise leg) • Diagnostic studies include X-rays and myelography.
• Predisposing factors include genetic history of scoliosis, poliomyelitis, congenital abnormalities.	• Limited range of motion; fatigued or tired back; hair patches, dimples, and pigmentation on back; decreased chest expansion; impaired pulmonary or cardiac function (hypoxia, cyanosis, chronic obstructive pulmonary disease); one scapula, breast, or flank more prominent than other; shoulders and hips not level • Diagnostic studies include X-rays.
• Compression fracture of thoracic vertebrae is a predisposing factor. • Recent spinal trauma, osteoporosis, chronic arthritis, tuberculosis	• Limited spinal range of motion; decreased pulmonary function • Diagnostic studies include X-rays.

Supportive-Structure Disorders

DISORDER	CHIEF COMPLAINTS
Spasmodic torticollis	• *Pain:* present with neck movement in trapezius, sternocleidomastoid, and other neck muscles; sudden or gradual onset; worsens under stress • *Joint stiffness:* stiff neck caused by muscle spasm • *Deformity and immobility:* muscle spasms cause head rotation to opposite side and flexion to same side
Bursitis	• *Pain:* severe on movement; in chronic form, nagging, intermittent pain possible • *Joint stiffness:* inflammation of bursae and calcific deposits in subdeltoid, olecranon (miners' elbow), trochanteric, or prepatellar (housemaid's knee) bursae. • *Swelling and redness:* over affected joint
Carpal tunnel syndrome	• *Pain:* worsens after manual activity or at night; radiates up arm; may be intermittent or constant • *Swelling and redness:* soft tissue swelling possible • *Deformity and immobility:* inability to oppose thumb and little finger • *Sensory changes:* numbness, burning, or tingling on palmar surface (may be initial symptom)

HISTORY	PHYSICAL EXAMINATION AND DIAGNOSTIC STUDIES
• Difficult birth is a predisposing factor. • Accompanying disorders include eye imbalance or defects, psychogenic problems, spinal or muscular defects. • Most common in adults ages 30 to 60	• Possible neck muscle spasms, which pull head forcibly to one side • Asymmetry of head and neck
• Predisposing factors include recent trauma to joint, occupational stress to joint, rheumatoid arthritis, gout, infection	• Decreased range of motion in affected joint
• Predisposing factors include trauma or injury to wrist, rheumatoid arthritis, gout, myxedema, diabetes mellitus, leukemia, acromegaly, edema associated with pregnancy. • Most common in postmenopausal women and in women in advanced pregnancy	• Atrophy of thenar eminences; positive Tinel's sign (tingling present with wrist percussion); positive Phalen's sign (tingling with sustained wrist flexion); muscle weakness; dryness of skin over thumb and first two fingers • Diagnostic studies may include electromyography.

Continued

Supportive-Structure Disorders
Continued

DISORDER	CHIEF COMPLAINTS
Tenosynovitis	• *Pain:* insidious or precipitated by strenuous activity; may radiate • *Joint stiffness:* joint locking possible; inflammation common • *Swelling and redness:* local swelling
Ganglion	• *Pain:* continuous aching aggravated by joint motion • *Joint stiffness:* present • *Swelling and redness:* gradual swelling over joint increased with extensive use of affected extremity; tense or fluctuant, rounded, nontender • *Deformity and immobility:* nodule over joint; weak fingers and joints next to ganglion, if connected to tendon sheath
Meniscal tear	• *Pain:* acute pain or localized tenderness • *Swelling and redness:* local swelling • *Deformity and immobility:* muscle atrophy of quadriceps muscle above knee; inability to straighten knee
Ligamental tear	• *Pain:* tenderness on palpation • *Joint stiffness:* sensation of slight catching • *Swelling and redness:* fluid around the joint, ecchymosis • *Deformity and immobility:* excessive tibia motion at anterior and posterior femur • *Sensory changes:* weakness, instability

OTHER BODY SYSTEM DISORDERS

HISTORY	PHYSICAL EXAMINATION AND DIAGNOSTIC STUDIES
• Predisposing factors include injury or surgery of involved joint. • Most common in women in early 40s	• Decreased range of motion; pain on palpation
• May occur after trauma, weight gain, compression • Disappears and recurs • Onset between adolescence and age 50 • Most common in women	• Limited range of motion of affected joint; palpable nodule more prominent on flexion, less prominent on extension
• Predisposing factors include twisting injury or direct blow to knee, repeated squatting or kneeling. • Most common in athletes	• Unequal knee contour; positive McMurray sign; blood in joint space
• Popping sound heard when injury occurred; trauma to knee • Most common in athletes	• Unstable knee joint; abnormal knee range of motion; point tenderness; changed knee joint contour

OTHER BODY SYSTEM DISORDERS

Continued

Supportive-Structure Disorders
Continued

DISORDER	CHIEF COMPLAINTS
Lower back strain	• *Pain:* acute and severe, or chronic, less severe, and aching; localized pain; may radiate • *Joint stiffness:* may be present • *Swelling and redness:* swelling caused by hemorrhage into tissues
Sprain	• *Pain:* varying degrees over involved joint • *Joint stiffness:* present • *Swelling and redness:* soft tissue swelling; superficial bruise • *Deformity and immobility:* limited range of motion • *Sensory changes:* can be seen in cervical sprain
Dislocation of the shoulder	• *Pain:* local, around involved joint • *Joint stiffness:* present; torn ligaments • *Swelling and redness:* soft tissue swelling • *Deformity and immobility:* displaced bones at joint; muscle atrophy

HISTORY	PHYSICAL EXAMINATION AND DIAGNOSTIC STUDIES
• Muscle suddenly forced beyond capacity; trauma; degenerative disk disease; continued mechanical strain; pregnancy	• Tenderness with firm pressure; bruise; muscle spasm; inflammation; decreased range of motion
• Sudden twisting injury	• Edema and discoloration around joint; no X-ray changes except soft tissue swelling; tenderness over joint
• Traumatic injury • Predisposing factors include congenital changes in skeletal contour, weakness of musculature, past history of dislocation • May reduce itself, or recur • Most common in young adults, athletes	• Decreased range of motion; altered joint configuration; changed extremity length

OTHER BODY SYSTEM DISORDERS

Muscular Function Disorders

DISORDER	CHIEF COMPLAINTS
Muscle cramp	• *Pain:* present; cause unknown • *Deformity and immobility:* immobility during cramp; deformity also present
Contractures	• *Pain:* absent • *Joint stiffness:* immobility caused by shortening of surrounding structures • *Deformity and immobility:* decreased mobility and function of affected part; deformity may result
Poliomyelitis	• *Pain:* headache; muscle stiffness; aching and pain; sore throat • *Joint stiffness:* stiff neck • *Deformity and immobility:* progressive motor paralysis • *Sensory changes:* occasional sensory changes
Limb-girdle dystrophy (Erb)	• *Deformity and immobility:* mild kyphoscoliosis possible; severe disability late in disease

HISTORY	PHYSICAL EXAMINATION AND DIAGNOSTIC STUDIES
• Common during pregnancy and in athletes • Usually occurs at night after strenuous activity	• Muscle is visibly and palpably tight; fasciculations; excessive sweating • Diagnostic studies include electromyography.
• Trauma, infection, nerve lesions, result of immobilization	• Shortening of skin, muscle, or ligaments; flexion of joint
• Most common in infants, children, and young adults • Usually occurs in midsummer or fall	• Low-grade fever; nausea, vomiting, diarrhea, constipation, muscles tender on palpation; diminished or absent deep tendon reflexes • Diagnostic studies include examination of spinal fluid.
• Most common in adults ages 20 to 30 • Inherited • Rate of progression and severity are variable	• Primarily involves shoulder and pelvic girdle muscles; peculiar gait; muscle weakness; muscle contractions; muscle fasciculations; occasionally pseudohypertrophy of other muscles; may lead to respiratory and cardiac muscle involvement • Diagnostic studies include muscle biopsy, serum enzymes, electromyography.

Clinical Effects of Sodium Imbalance

Sodium is the major cation (90%) in extracellular fluid; potassium, the major cation in intracellular fluid. During repolarization, the sodium-potassium pump continually shifts sodium into the cells and potassium out of the cells; during depolarization, it does the reverse. Sodium cation functions include maintaining tonicity and concentration of extracellular fluid, acid-base balance (reabsorption of sodium ion and excretion of hydrogen ion), nerve conduction and neuromuscular function, glandular secretion and water balance. Although the body requires only 2 to 4 g of sodium daily, most Americans consume 6 to 10 g daily (mostly sodium chloride, as table salt), excreting excess sodium through the kidneys and skin.

A low-sodium diet or excessive use of diuretics may induce hyponatremia (decreased serum sodium concentration); dehydration may induce hypernatremia (increased serum sodium concentration).

Normal sodium plasma value: 136 to 145 mEq/liter

DYSFUNCTION	HYPONATREMIA	HYPERNATREMIA
CNS	• Anxiety, head-aches, muscle twitching and weakness, seizures	• Fever, agitation, restlessness, seizures
Cardiovascular	• Hypotension; tachycardia; with severe deficit, vasomotor collapse, thready pulse	• Hypertension, tachycardia, pitting edema, excessive weight gain
Gastrointestinal	• Nausea, vomiting, abdominal cramps	• Rough, dry tongue; intense thirst
Genitourinary	• Oliguria or anuria	• Oliguria
Respiratory	• Cyanosis with severe deficiency	• Dyspnea, respiratory arrest, and death (from dramatic rise in osmotic pressure)
Cutaneous	• Cold clammy skin, decreased skin turgor	• Flushed skin; dry, sticky mucous membranes

Clinical Features of Potassium Imbalance

Normal potassium plasma value: 3.5 to 5.0 mEq/liter

DYSFUNCTION	HYPOKALEMIA	HYPERKALEMIA
Cardiovascular	• Dizziness, hypotension, dysrhythmias, EKG changes (flattened T waves, elevated U waves, depressed ST segment), cardiac arrest (with serum potassium levels < 2.5 mEq/liter)	• Tachycardia and later bradycardia, EKG changes (tented and elevated T waves, widened QRS, prolonged PR interval, flattened or absent P waves, depressed ST segment), cardiac arrest (with levels > 7.0 mEq/liter)
Gastrointestinal	• Nausea and vomiting, anorexia, diarrhea, abdominal distention, paralytic ileus or decreased peristalsis	• Nausea, diarrhea, abdominal cramps
Musculoskeletal	• Muscle weakness and fatigue, leg cramps	• Muscle weakness, flaccid paralysis
Genitourinary	• Polyuria	• Oliguria, anuria
CNS	• Malaise, irritability, confusion, mental depression, speech changes, decreased reflexes, respiratory paralysis	• Hyperreflexia progressing to weakness, numbness, tingling, and flaccid paralysis
Acid-base balance	• Metabolic alkalosis	• Metabolic acidosis

OTHER BODY SYSTEM DISORDERS

Symptoms of Calcium Imbalance

Normal calcium plasma value: 4.5 to 5.5 mEq/liter or 8.8 to 10.5 mg/ 100 ml

DYSFUNCTION	HYPOCALCEMIA	HYPERCALCEMIA
CNS	• Anxiety, irritability, twitching around mouth, laryngospasm, convulsions, Chvostek's sign, Trousseau's sign	• Drowsiness, lethargy, headaches, depression or apathy, irritability, confusion
Musculoskeletal	• Paresthesia (tingling and numbness), tetany or painful tonic muscle spasms, facial spasms, abdominal cramps, muscle cramps, spasmodic contractions	• Weakness, muscle flaccidity, bone pain, pathologic fractures
Cardiovascular	• Dysrhythmias, hypotension	• Signs of heart block, cardiac arrest in systole, hypertension
Gastrointestinal	• Increased GI motility, diarrhea	• Anorexia, nausea, vomiting, constipation, dehydration, polydipsia
Other	• Blood-clotting abnormalities	• Renal polyuria, flank pain, and, eventually, azotemia

Signs and Symptoms of Magnesium Imbalance

Approximately one third of magnesium taken into the body is absorbed through the small intestine and is eventually excreted in urine; the remaining unabsorbed magnesium is excreted in stool.

Since many common foods contain magnesium, a dietary deficiency is rare. Magnesium deficiency (hypomagnesemia) generally follows impaired absorption or too rapid excretion of magnesium. It frequently coexists with other electrolyte imbalances, especially low calcium and potassium levels. Magnesium excess (hypermagnesemia) is common in patients with renal failure and excessive intake of magnesium-containing antacids.

Normal magnesium plasma value: 1.5 to 2.5 mEq/liter

DYSFUNCTION	HYPOMAGNESEMIA	HYPERMAGNESEMIA
Neuromuscular	• Hyperirritability, tetany, leg and foot cramps, Chvostek's sign (facial muscle spasms induced by tapping the branches of the facial nerve)	• Diminished reflexes, muscle weakness, flaccid paralysis, respiratory muscle paralysis that may cause respiratory distress
CNS	• Confusion, delusions, hallucinations, convulsions	• Drowsiness, flushing, lethargy, confusion, diminished sensorium
Cardiovascular	• Dysrhythmias, vasomotor changes (vasodilation and hypotension), occasionally, hypertension	• Bradycardia, weak pulse, hypotension, heart block, cardiac arrest (with serum levels of 25 mEq/liter)

Guide to Nutritional Disorders

MARASMUS (nonedematous protein-calorie malnutrition)

Chief complaints
- *Weight change:* loss may be profound
- *Skin changes:* dryness
- *Asthenia:* usually present; if severe, can result in profound weakness
- *Gastrointestinal problems:* frequent diarrhea
- *Musculoskeletal impairment:* growth retardation in children; muscular wasting

History
- Inadequate intake of proteins and calories; may occur in hospitalized patients with conditions such as cancer, Crohn's disease, and cirrhosis

Physical examination
- Weight/height ratio 60% to 90% below standard; triceps skinfold thickness usually 60% below standard; mid–upper-arm circumference and mid–upper-arm muscle circumference usually 60% to 90% below normal

Diagnostic studies
- Decreased plasma albumin
- Electrolyte depletion, especially potassium and magnesium
- Iron deficiency anemia
- Decreased BUN

KWASHIORKOR (edematous protein-calorie malnutrition)

Chief complaints
- *Weight loss:* loss may be profound
- *Skin changes:* dry and peeling
- *Nails:* spoon-shaped and brittle
- *Hair:* dull, sparse, and dry
- *Asthenia:* usually present
- *Gastrointestinal problems:* anorexia and diarrhea are common; nausea and vomiting may be present
- *Musculoskeletal impairment:* severe muscle wasting often masked by edema

History
- Common in underdeveloped countries and in areas where dietary amino acid content is insufficient for growth requirements
- Typically occurs at about age 1, after infants are weaned from breast milk to a protein-deficient diet of starchy gruels or sugar water, but it can develop at any time during the formative years.

Physical examination
- Normal height, but weight less than 80% of standard for the patient's age and sex, below standard arm circumference and triceps skinfold; protruding abdomen; hepatomegaly; vital signs: low temperature, slow pulse and respirations

Continued

Guide to Nutritional Disorders
Continued

KWASHIORKOR
Continued

Diagnostic studies
• Serum albumin less than 2.8 g/ 100 ml; positive reactions to skin tests; moderate anemia

OBESITY

Chief complaints
• *Weight change:* significant gain over time
• *Skin changes:* thick, pale striae
• *Asthenia:* may be present
• *Gastrointestinal problems:* none obviously related
• *Musculoskeletal impairment:* possible joint strain or pain
History
• Pattern of overeating, decreased energy expenditure, endocrine abnormality
Physical examination
• Weight/height ratio 20% or more above normal, triceps skinfold measurement indicating obesity
Diagnostic studies
• None significant

VITAMIN A DEFICIENCY

Chief complaints
• *Weight change:* none
• *Skin changes:* dry, scaly, roughness with follicular hyperkeratosis; shrinking and hardening of mucous membranes
• *Asthenia:* vague apathy may be present
• *Gastrointestinal problems:* none
• *Musculoskeletal impairment:* possible failure to thrive
History
• Night blindness that may progress to permanent blindness; diet lacking in leafy green and yellow fruits and vegetables; fat malabsorption
Physical examination
• Dryness, roughness of conjunctiva; swelling and redness of lids; clouded cornea; ulcerations possible
Diagnostic studies
• Serum values for vitamin A below 20 mcg/100 ml confirm deficiency.

THIAMINE (B₁) DEFICIENCY

Chief complaints
• *Weight change:* emaciated appearance in dry form
• *Skin changes:* pallor; edema in wet form
• *Asthenia:* apathy and confusion, loss of memory
• *Gastrointestinal problems:* anorexia, vomiting, constipation, abdominal pain may occur
• *Musculoskeletal impairment:* muscle cramps, paresthesias, polyneuritis; seizures, paralysis, muscular atrophy

Continued

OTHER BODY SYSTEM DISORDERS

Guide to Nutritional Disorders
Continued

THIAMINE (B₁) DEFICIENCY
Continued

History
• Fever; pregnancy; inadequate intake of whole-grain or enriched breads or cereals, pork, beans, and nuts; malabsorption syndrome; chronic alcoholism
Physical examination
• In wet form, edema begins in legs and progresses upward. Cardiomegaly with tachycardia, dyspnea may occur; nystagmus possible; hyperactive knee-jerk reflex, followed by hypoactivity
Diagnostic studies
• Serum values for thiamine less than 5 mcg/100 ml; elevated levels of pyruvic and lactic acid; low urine values for thiamine; nonspecific EKG changes

RIBOFLAVIN (B₂) DEFICIENCY

Chief complaints
• *Weight change:* less common
• *Skin changes:* seborrheic dermatitis in the nasolabial folds, scrotum, and vulva; generalized dermatitis
• *Asthenia:* usually present
• *Gastrointestinal problems:* not common
• *Musculoskeletal impairment:* possible growth retardation
History
• Inadequate intake of milk, meat, fish, leafy green and yellow vegetables; chronic alcoholism; use of oral contraceptives
Physical examination
• Cheilosis, conjunctivitis in mild form; in late stages, moderate edema, neuropathy
Diagnostic studies
• Riboflavin serum level less than 2 mcg/100 ml; prolonged diarrhea; complaints of photophobia and itching, burning, tearing eyes

NIACIN DEFICIENCY

Chief complaints
• *Weight change:* loss possible, even in early stages
• *Skin changes:* mild eruptions in early stage, progressing to scaly dermatitis resembling severe sunburn
• *Asthenia:* present; fatigue even in early stages
• *Gastrointestinal problems:* anorexia, indigestion, nausea, vomiting, diarrhea possible
• *Musculoskeletal impairment:* muscle weakness in early stages; growth retardation in children in late-stage deficiency
History
• Inadequate intake of niacin, especially where corn is staple food; secondary to carcinoid syndrome or Hartnup disease, chronic alcoholism

Continued

Guide to Nutritional Disorders
Continued

NIACIN DEFICIENCY
Continued

Physical examination
• Mouth, tongue, and lips become reddened; atrophy of papillae; in late stages, confusion and disorientation
Diagnostic studies
• Serum niacin levels less than 30 mcg/100 ml; headache, backache, sore mouth

VITAMIN C DEFICIENCY

Chief complaints
• *Weight change:* loss possible
• *Skin changes:* drying roughness and dingy brown color change; petechiae, ecchymosis, follicular hyperkeratosis
• *Gastrointestinal problems:* anorexia, diarrhea, vomiting possible in children
• *Musculoskeletal impairment:* limb and joint pain and swelling
History
• Inadequate intake of fresh fruits and vegetables; overcooking; marginal intake during periods of stress. Groups at risk include infants fed processed cow's milk only, those on limited diets, and those with bizarre eating habits.
Physical examination
• Swollen and/or bleeding gums (early sign), loosening of teeth,

pallor, ocular hemorrhages in the bulbar conjunctivas; delayed wound healing and tissue repair
Diagnostic studies
• Serum ascorbic acid levels less than 0.4 mg/100 ml and WBC ascorbic acid levels less than 25 mg/100 ml (help confirm); poor wound healing; psychologic disturbances, such as hysteria, depression, anemia

VITAMIN D DEFICIENCY

Chief complaints
• *Weight change:* none
• *Skin changes:* none
• *Asthenia:* not present
• *Gastrointestinal problems:* none
• *Musculoskeletal impairment:* chronic deficiency causes bone malformations from bone softening and retarded growth
History
• Inadequate dietary intake of vitamin D; malabsorption; inadequate exposure to sunlight; hepatic or renal disease
Physical examination
• Characteristic bone malformations
Diagnostic studies
• Plasma calcium levels less than 7.5 mg/100 ml; inorganic phosphorus serum levels less than 3 mg/100 ml; serum citrate levels less than 2.5 mg/100 ml

Continued

Guide to Nutritional Disorders
Continued

VITAMIN K DEFICIENCY

Chief complaints
• *Weight change:* none
• *Skin changes:* petechiae and ecchymosis possible
• *Asthenia:* present; may be related to blood loss
• *Gastrointestinal problems:* gastrointestinal bleeding, which can include massive hemorrhage, possible
• *Musculoskeletal impairment:* hemorrhaging in muscles, joints
History
• Prolonged use of such drugs as anticoagulants and antibiotics; malabsorption of vitamin K (as in sprue, bowel resection, ulcerative colitis), biliary obstruction
Physical examination
• Bleeding tendencies
Diagnostic studies
• Prolonged prothrombin time (25% longer than control)

IRON DEFICIENCY

Chief complaints
• *Weight change:* none
• *Skin changes:* pallor
• *Asthenia:* present; may be extreme in severe cases

• *Gastrointestinal problems:* anorexia, flatulence, epigastric distress, constipation
• *Musculoskeletal impairment:* numbness, tingling of extremities; neuralgic pain possible
History
• Inadequate dietary intake of iron as prolonged unsupplemented breast- or bottle-feeding or in periods of stress; iron malabsorption, such as in diarrhea, gastrectomy, celiac disease; blood loss
Physical examination
• In chronic form: nails become brittle, spoon-shaped; corners of the mouth crack, tongue becomes smooth; in severe cases: tachycardia, dyspnea on exertion, listlessness, irritability; liver and spleen enlargement possible
Diagnostic studies
• Low hemoglobin, less than 12 g/100 ml for males, less than 10 g/100 ml for females; low hematocrit, less than 47 ml/100 ml for males, less than 42 ml/100 for females; low serum iron levels with high binding capacity; low serum ferritin levels

Continued

Guide to Nutritional Disorders
Continued

IODINE DEFICIENCY

Chief complaints
• *Weight change:* none
• *Skin changes:* dry, cold skin in severe stages
• *Asthenia:* present; may occur even in mild deficiency
• *Gastrointestinal problems:* anorexia
• *Musculoskeletal impairment:* none

History
• Insufficient intake (table salt, seafood); increased metabolic demands (growth, pregnancy, lactation)
• Poor memory, chills, menorrhagia, amenorrhea

Physical examination
• Hoarseness, hearing loss, thick tongue, bradycardia, lowered blood pressure, delayed relaxation phase in deep tendon reflexes
• Mild deficiency may produce lassitude, fatigue, and loss of motivation; severe deficiency generates overt and often unmistakable features of hypothyroidism, such as hoarseness, thick tongue, hearing loss, anorexia, poor memory, weakness, bradycardia, and decreased cardiac output

Diagnostic studies
• Low T_4 with high ^{131}I uptake, low 24-hour urine iodine, and high TSH. T_3 or T_4 resin uptake test shows values 25% below normal.

FOLIC ACID DEFICIENCY ANEMIA

Chief complaints
• *Weight change:* loss common
• *Skin changes:* severe pallor
• *Fatigue:* progressive; asthenia
• *Gastrointestinal problems:* diarrhea, nausea, anorexia, jaundice
• *Musculoskeletal impairment:* absent
• *Respiratory changes:* shortness of breath
• *Neurologic changes:* headache, fainting, irritability, and forgetfulness

History
• Inadequate intake of leafy vegetables, organ meats, beef, wheat. Most common in infants, pregnant women, chronic alcoholics, and patients with malabsorption disorders

Physical examination
• Glossitis, cardiac enlargement, macrocytic megaloblastic anemia

Diagnostic studies
• Serum value less than 100 ng/ml

Continued

OTHER BODY SYSTEM DISORDERS

Guide to Nutritional Disorders
Continued

VITAMIN B$_{12}$ DEFICIENCY

Chief complaints
• *Weight change:* loss possible
• *Skin changes:* lemon-yellow pallor
• *Asthenia:* present
• *Gastrointestinal problems:* anorexia, vomiting, diarrhea
• *Musculoskeletal impairment:* Hand and foot paresthesia; degeneration of spinal cord, decreased musculoskeletal innervation

History
• Strict vegetarian; malabsorption resulting from gastrectomy or ileal resection

Physical examination
• Macrocytic megaloblastic anemia, bright red tongue, cardiovascular changes, dyspnea, chest pain, chronic congestive heart failure

Diagnostic studies
• Serum value less than 100 pg/ml; resembles folic acid deficiency, with additional neural and mental changes

VITAMIN E DEFICIENCY

Chief complaint
• *Skin changes:* edema and skin lesions in infants, erythematous papular skin eruption followed by desquamation in premature infants

• *Musculoskeletal impairment:* muscle weakness or intermittent claudication in adults

History
• Mainly seen in low birth weight or premature infants, uncommon in adults
• Deficiency develops in conditions associated with fat malabsorption, such as kwashiorkor, celiac disease, or cystic fibrosis

Physical examination
• Difficult to recognize but usually shows signs and symptoms of hemolytic anemia

Diagnostic studies
• Serum alpha-tocopherol levels below 0.5 mg/100 ml, excessive creatinuria, increased creatine phosphokinase, hemolytic anemia, elevated platelet count

ANOREXIA NERVOSA

Chief complaints
• *Weight loss:* weight loss for no organic reason
• *Skin changes:* chronic undernourishment, loss of fatty tissue, blotchy or sallow skin, lanugo on the face and body
• *Hair:* dryness or loss of scalp hair
• *Teeth:* dental caries

Continued

Guide to Nutritional Disorders
Continued

ANOREXIA NERVOSA
Continued

- *Gastrointestinal problems:* gorging followed by spontaneous or self-induced vomiting or self-administration of laxatives or diuretics, dehydration, constipation.
- *Genitourinary problems:* amenorrhea
- *Cardiovascular problems:* hypotension, dysrhythmias
- *Musculoskeletal impairment:* skeletal muscle atrophy
- *Psychological problems:* morbid dread of being fat, shows a compulsion to being thin, may be obsessed with food, but refuses to eat
- *Miscellaneous:* intolerance to cold, susceptibility to infection
History
- Self-imposed starvation. Gorging, vomiting, and purging may occur during starvation or after normal weight is restored as a means of weight control.
- Primarily affects adolescent females and young adults
- A higher rate of attempted suicides occurs with these patients.
Physical examination
- Weight loss of 20% or more, undernourishment, emaciation
Diagnostic studies
- Laboratory data is usually normal unless weight loss exceeds 30%

BULIMIA

Chief complaints
- *Weight changes:* frequent fluctuations, but weight may be within a normal range
- *Teeth:* dental caries, gum infections
- *Gastrointestinal problems:* binge eating may be followed by purging (self-induced vomiting) or self-administration of laxatives or diuretics; dehydration possible.
- *Psychological problems:* depressive behavior may be seen along with overwhelming obsession with food, compulsion to eat.
History
- Episodes of binge eating (usually sweet, high-caloric content, and soft foods) that may be followed by purging.
- Primarily affects adolescent females and young adults
- Various psychosocial factors may contribute to its development.
Physical examination
- Fluctuation in weight, otherwise may be nonspecific.
Diagnostic studies
- Laboratory data may indicate electrolyte imbalance.

Identifying Third-Space Edema

ANASARCA (GENERALIZED MASSIVE EDEMA)

Signs and symptoms
- Increase in pitting edema values
- Progressive increase in extremity circumference

Treatment
- Determine cause and correct it, if possible. (May be associated with end-stage kidney disease or cancer.)
- Administer mannitol or albumin I.V., as ordered. *Note:* Give other diuretics with caution.
- Restrict fluid and salt intake, as ordered.
- Give analgesics, as ordered.

Special considerations
- Elevate dependent body parts.
- Turn patient frequently; massage sacrum, hips, and other affected body areas.
- If patient's face is affected, warn him that his eyes may swell shut.
- If his neck is affected, frequently check for a compromised airway. Keep a tracheotomy tray on hand.
- Remove rings, bracelets, or tight clothing. Make sure the patient's identification bracelet is nonconstrictive.
- Don't give injections in edematous areas.

COMPARTMENT SYNDROME (MUSCLE COMPARTMENT EDEMA)

Signs and symptoms
- Increase in pitting edema values
- Increase in extremity circumference
- Cool skin distal to compartment
- Possible sensation loss

Treatment
- Determine cause and correct it, if possible.
- Give analgesics, as ordered.

Special considerations
- Promote venous and lymphatic draining by keeping extremity at heart level.
- Remove rings, bracelets, and tight clothing.
- Measure extremity circumference at least every 2 hours.
- Monitor compartment pressure with pressure monitoring equipment, if ordered.
- Periodically, check patient's pulses, color, temperature, and capillary refill distal to edema.
- Don't give injections in edematous areas.

  Note: If edema compromises vascular and nerve supply to the affected area, the doctor may perform a fasciotomy. Prepare the patient for this procedure, if indicated.

Continued

Identifying Third-Space Edema
Continued

HYDROPERICARDITIS (PERI-
CARDIAL EDEMA)

Signs and symptoms
- Pericardial friction rub
- Progressive increase in central venous pressure (CVP)
- Enlarged heart on chest X-ray
- Jugular vein distention
- Faint heart sounds possible
- Dyspnea
- Orthopnea
- Tachycardia

Treatment
- Determine cause and correct it, if possible.
- Keep patient on bed rest to reduce cardiac demand.
- Give oxygen and analgesics, if ordered.
- If indicated, prepare patient for invasive treatment; for example, partial pericardectomy (which allows fluid to flow into the pleural space) or fluid aspiration with cardiac needle

Special considerations
- Keep cardiac needle and large syringe handy. Edema may cause pericardial compression.
- Monitor vital signs at least every 30 minutes.
- Monitor for CVP increase (caused by compression of

heart's right side).
- Auscultate to detect friction rub.

PLEURAL EFFUSION (EDEMA
IN PLEURAL SPACE)

Signs and symptoms
- Decreased breath sounds
- Absent or diminished voice sounds
- Dullness over affected area on percussion
- Pleuritic chest pain; may radiate to neck, shoulders, or abdomen
- Dyspnea
- Shortness of breath
- Poorly defined intercostal space on affected side
- Tachycardia
- Displaced heart sounds
- Gallop heart rhythms
- Hypoxia

Treatment
- Correct cause, if possible.
- Give oxygen, as ordered.

Special considerations
- Monitor arterial blood gas measurements.
- Encourage deep breathing to prevent atelectasis.
- If condition is severe, prepare patient for chest tube insertion or thoracentesis.
- Discourage smoking

Continued

Identifying Third-Space Edema
Continued

PULMONARY EDEMA

Signs and symptoms
- Enlarged heart and congested pulmonary vessels on chest X-ray
- Shortness of breath
- Pink, frothy sputum
- Crackles on auscultation
- Orthopnea
- Tachycardia
- Coughing
- Tachypnea

Treatment
- Support respiration and give oxygen, as needed.
- Give bronchodilators, such as aminophylline, as ordered.
- Give diuretics, such as furosemide (Lasix*) or ethacrynic acid (Edecrin*), as ordered.
- If ordered, give morphine sulfate.
- If ordered, give digitalis.
  Note: As an emergency measure, the doctor may order rotating tourniquets to reduce blood volume returning to the heart.

Special considerations
- Monitor vital signs hourly.
- Place patient in high Fowler's position.
- Monitor arterial blood gases.
- Prepare patient for rotating tourniquets, if ordered.

*Available in both the United States and Canada

ASCITES (ABDOMINAL EDEMA)

Signs and symptoms
- Increased abdominal girth
- Umbilicus extroversion
- Prominent abdominal veins

Treatment
- Determine cause and correct it, if possible.
- Increase intravascular osmotic pressure by administering albumin I.V., as ordered. Increased osmotic pressure helps draw fluid from the third space into the blood vessels, for elimination by the kidneys.
- Administer diuretics cautiously. Diuretics rapidly decrease intravascular volume (possibly causing hypovolemia) but have little or no effect on ascites.
- Restrict fluid intake, as ordered.
- Provide oxygen, if ordered.

Special considerations
- Assess for numbness and tingling of lower extremities from pressure on inferior vena cava.
- Place patient in semi-Fowler's position or help him sit upright in a chair to relieve pressure on his diaphragm.
- If indicated, prepare patient for invasive treatment; for example, LeVeen shunt insertion to allow one-way flow of ascites fluid from abdomen to the superior vena cava.

Complications of Intravenous Hyperalimentation

CONDITION/CAUSE	SIGNS AND SYMPTOMS	TREATMENT
Hyperglycemia Too rapid IVH delivery rate, lowered glucose tolerance, excessive total dextrose load	Glycosuria, nausea, vomiting, diarrhea, confusion, headache, and lethargy; untreated hyperosmolar hyperglycemic dehydration can lead to seizures, coma, and death.	Add insulin to the IVH solution.
Hypoglycemia Excess endogenous insulin production after abrupt termination of IVH solution, or excessive delivery of exogenous insulin	Muscle weakness, anxiety, confusion, restlessness, diaphoresis, vertigo, pallor, tremors, and palpitations	If possible, give carbohydrates orally; infuse dextrose 10% in water, or administer dextrose 50% in water by I.V. bolus.
Fluid deficit Hyperglycemia, vomiting, diarrhea, fistula output, large burns, inadequate fluid replacement, electrolyte imbalance	Fatigue, dry skin, and mucous membranes, lengthwise wrinkles in tongue, tachycardia, tachypnea, decreased urinary output, decreased central venous pressure, acute weight loss, hemoconcentration	Increase fluid intake.
Fluid excess Fluid overload, electrolyte imbalance	Puffy eyelids, peripheral edema, elevated central venous pressure, ascites, acute weight gain, pulmonary edema, pleural effusion, moist rales	Decrease fluid intake.

OTHER BODY SYSTEM DISORDERS

Continued

Complications of Intravenous Hyperalimentation
Continued

CONDITION/ CAUSE	SIGNS AND SYMPTOMS	TREATMENT
Hypokalemia Muscle catabolism, prolonged vomiting or suction, diarrhea; may occur when anabolism is achieved, with its accompanying intracellular movement of potassium	Malaise, lethargy, loss of deep tendon reflexes, muscle cramping, paresthesia, atrial and ventricular dysrhythmias, decreased intensity of heart sounds, weak pulse, hypotension, and complete heart block	Increase potassium intake. Malnourished patient may require an initial dose of 60 to 100 mEq/1,000 calories.
Hypophosphatemia Phosphate deficiency; infusion of glucose	Serum PO_4 levels < 1 mg/dl cause lethargy, weakness, paresthesia, glucose intolerance. Severe hypophosphatemia can cause acute hemolytic anemia, seizures, coma, and death.	Add phosphates to the IVH solution.
Hypocalcemia Increased doses of phosphates administered to correct hypophosphatemia, without supplemental calcium; may also result from hypoalbuminemia or excess free water	Nausea, vomiting, diarrhea, hyperactive reflexes, tingling at fingertips and mouth, carpopedal spasm, dysrhythmias, tetany, and convulsions	Add calcium to the IVH solution.

OTHER BODY SYSTEM DISORDERS

Continued

Complications of Intravenous Hyperalimentation
Continued

CONDITION/ CAUSE	SIGNS AND SYMPTOMS	TREATMENT
Hypomagnesemia Inadequate intake of magnesium; severe diarrhea and vomiting	Lethargy, tremors, positive Chvostek's sign or Trousseau's sign, painful paresthesia, convulsions, and tetany	Add magnesium to the IVH solution.
Essential fatty acid deficiency Absent or inadequate fat intake for an extended period	Alopecia, brittle nails, dermatitis, increased capillary fragility, indolent wound healing, reduced prostaglandin synthesis, increased platelet aggregation, thrombocytopenia, enhanced susceptibility to infection, fatty liver infiltration, lipid accumulation in pulmonary macrophages, notching of R waves on EKG	For the adult patient, infuse two or three bottles of 10% or 20% fat emulsions daily.
Zinc deficiency Altered requirements associated with stress, the degree of intracellular zinc deficit, and induced zinc deficiencies from redistribution during the anabolism	Diarrhea, apathy, confusion, depression, eczema, alopecia, decreased libido, hypogonadism, indolent wound healing, acute growth arrest, hyperpigmentation, soft and misshapen nails, anorexia, hypogeusethesia (decreased taste acuity), dysgeusia (unpleasant taste), hyposmia (decreased odor acuity), dysomia (unpleasant odor in nasopharynx), iron deficiency anemia, and bone deformities	Add zinc to the IVH solution.

Continued

OTHER BODY SYSTEM DISORDERS

Complications of Intravenous Hyperalimentation
Continued

CONDITION/ CAUSE	SIGNS AND SYMPTOMS	TREATMENT
Hypocupremia Long-term administration of IVH without addition of copper sulfate; infection, high-output enterocutaneous fistulas, and diarrhea.	Neutropenia and hypochromic and microcytic anemia	Add copper to the IVH solution.

Ambulatory Hyperalimentation Vest

The ambulatory hyperalimentation vest, illustrated below, allows continuous delivery of parenteral nutrition without restricting the patient's mobility.

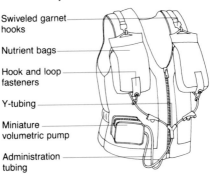

Swiveled garnet hooks

Nutrient bags

Hook and loop fasteners

Y-tubing

Miniature volumetric pump

Administration tubing

Bacterial and Viral Diseases

SCARLET FEVER

Chief complaints
- *Itching:* absent
- *Rash:* present; bright red, finely papular in skin creases of axillae, groin, and neck; spreads rapidly to trunk, extremities, and face; lasts 1 or 2 days

History
- Exposure to infected person 1 or 2 days previously
- Accompanied by sore throat, headache, vomiting

Physical examination and diagnostic studies
- Red pharynx, with exudate
- Strawberry red tongue
- Fever
- Peeling skin on hands and feet possible after several days.

IMPETIGO

Chief complaints
- *Itching:* present
- *Rash:* small, very fragile vesicles; when broken, exudes liquid that dries and forms honey-colored crusts; usually occurs on face

History
- Most common in children during hot weather
- Predisposing factors: overcrowded living quarters, poor skin hygiene, anemia, malnutrition, minor skin trauma

Physical examination and diagnostic studies
- Culture and sensitivity tests show *Streptococcus pyogenes* and *Staphylococcus aureus.*

HERPES SIMPLEX TYPE 1 (FEVER BLISTER)

Chief complaints
- *Itching:* absent
- *Rash:* present; single group of vesicles ruptures, leaving a painful ulcer, followed by a yellow crust; usually occurs around mouth or nose but may occur anywhere on body; healing begins 7 to 10 days after initial onset, is complete within 3 weeks
- *Lesion:* absent

History
- Cold, fever, trauma, menstruation, or overexposure to sunlight may occur prior to sores.
- Recurrences common

Physical examination and diagnostic studies
- No other physical characteristics

HERPES PROGENITALIS TYPE 2 (HERPES SIMPLEX)

Chief complaints
- *Itching:* absent
- *Rash:* present; small-grouped

Continued

Bacterial and Viral Diseases
Continued

HERPES PROGENITALIS TYPE
2 (HERPES SIMPLEX)
Continued

vesicles around genital and mouth
areas
• *Lesion:* absent
History
• *In infants:* delivered vaginally
from infected mother
• *In adolescents and adults:* sex-
ual contact with infected person
**Physical examination and diag-
nostic studies**
• No other physical characteris-
tics

HERPES ZOSTER (SHINGLES)

Chief complaints
• *Itching:* absent
• *Rash:* present; grouped vesicles
or crusted lesions along nerve
root, usually unilateral
• *Lesion:* absent
History
• Chicken pox
• Persistent postherpetic neural-
gia possible
**Physical examination and diag-
nostic studies**
• No other physical characteris-
tics

RUBEOLA (MEASLES)

Chief complaints
• *Itching:* absent

• *Rash:* present; begins with faint
macules on hairline, neck, and
cheeks; increases to maculopapular rash on entire face, neck, and
upper arms; spreads to back, abdomen, arms, thighs, and lower
legs; appears 2 to 4 days after
onset of other symptoms; lasts 4
or 5 days
• *Lesion:* absent
History
• Exposure to infected person 10
to 14 days previously
• Cold, conjunctivitis, fever, and
cough prior to rash
• Greatest communicability 11
days after exposure, lasting 4 or 5
days
**Physical examination and diag-
nostic studies**
• Koplik's spots (white patches on
oral mucosa)
• Generalized lymphadenopathy,
conjunctivitis

RUBELLA (GERMAN MEASLES)

Chief complaints
• *Itching:* absent
• *Rash:* present; begins with
maculopapular rash on face,
which spreads to trunk
• *Lesion:* absent
History
• Exposure to infected person 14
to 21 days previously
• *In children:* usually no symp-
toms prior to rash   *Continued*

Bacterial and Viral Diseases
Continued

RUBELLA (GERMAN MEASLES)
Continued

- *In adolescents:* headache, malaise, anorexia may occur prior to rash

Physical examination and diagnostic studies
- *In adolescents and adults:* conjunctivitis, low-grade fever, posterior cervical and postauricular lymphadenopathy, joint pain

EXANTHEMA SUBITUM (ROSEOLA INFANTUM)

Chief complaints
- *Itching:* present
- *Rash:* present; begins with macular or maculopapular eruption on trunk; *rarely* spreads to arms, neck, face, and legs; fades within 24 hours
- *Lesion:* absent

History
- Exposure to infected person 7 to 17 days previously
- Sudden high fever 3 or 4 days prior to rash
- Usually affects infants and children age 6 months to 3 years

Physical examination and diagnostic studies
- Inflamed pharynx

VARICELLA (CHICKEN POX)

Chief complaints
- *Itching:* present; urticaria around vesicle
- *Rash:* present; begins with crops of small red papules and clear vesicles on red base; vesicles break and then dry, causing crust formation; begins on trunk and spreads to face and scalp
- *Lesion:* present; may leave scars

History
- Exposure to infected person 13 to 21 days previously
- Malaise, anorexia prior to rash
- In temperate areas, higher incidence in later fall, winter, and spring

Physical examination and diagnostic studies
- Slight fever
- Palpation: enlarged lymph nodes
- Culture of V-2 virus
- Complement fixation positive for V-2 antibody
- Multinucleated, giant epithelial cells visible on microscopic examination of skin lesion scrapings

INDEX

INDEX

INDEX

INDEX